Natural Baby Care

Natural Baby Care

raising your child the way nature intended

Kim Davies

southwater

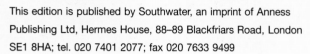

This edition is published by Southwater, an imprint of Anness Publishing Ltd, Hermes House, 88–89 Blackfriars Road, London SE1 8HA; tel. 020 7401 2077; fax 020 7633 9499

www.southwaterbooks.com; www.annesspublishing.com

If you like the images in this book and would like to investigate using them for publishing, promotions or advertising, please visit our website www.practicalpictures.com for more information.

UK agent: The Manning Partnership Ltd; tel. 01225 478444; fax 01225 478440; sales@manning-partnership.co.uk
UK distributor: Grantham Book Services Ltd; tel. 01476 541080; fax 01476 541061; orders@gbs.tbs-ltd.co.uk
North American agent/distributor: National Book Network; tel. 301 459 3366; fax 301 429 5746; www.nbnbooks.com
Australian agent/distributor: Pan Macmillan Australia; tel. 1300 135 113; fax 1300 135 103; customer.service@macmillan.com.au
New Zealand agent/distributor: David Bateman Ltd; tel. (09) 415 7664; fax (09) 415 8892

Publisher: Joanna Lorenz
Editorial Director: Helen Sudell
Executive Editor: Joanne Rippin
Designer: Nigel Partridge
Jacket Design: Lisa Tai
Photographer: Scott Morrison
Artworks: Anthony Duke

Photographs also taken by: Jo Harrison: 51tl, 65tm, 66b, 69t, 93b, 107t, 109t, 112b, 115tr, 119tl.

Thank you to the parents and children who appear in the photos: Achael and Amelia Brimson, Alfonso Perez, Andrea and Kiera Thompson, Andrew, Catherine and Scarlett Gordon, Beth and Owen Pierce, Christine and Grace Lewis, Elizabeth and Oliver Allen, Evie and Billie Beswick, Hazel and Isaac Plowman, Irena and Rose Andrews, Jancien and Arabella Lambeth, Marion Demoissier and Louisa Swann.

Thanks to the following agencies for supplying additional images: Alamy: 14rm, 36t & bl, 39tr, 50t, 59tl, 62t, 63t (both), 66t, 67tr, 82b, 102t, 108t, 110, 111 both, 114 both, 116, 121 tr, 141tr, 146b, 150t.
Corbis: pp13tr, 23tr, 41tr, 65br, 92bl.
The Science Photo Library: p47bl.

ETHICAL TRADING POLICY
Because of our ongoing ecological investment programme, you, as our customer, can have the pleasure and reassurance of knowing that a tree is being cultivated on your behalf to naturally replace the materials used to make the book you are holding. For further information about this scheme, go to www.annesspublishing.com/trees.

Previously published as part of a larger volume: *Baby and Childcare*

The author and publishers have made every effort to ensure that all instructions contained within this book are accurate and safe, and cannot accept liability for any resulting injury, damage or loss to persons or property, however it may arise. If you or your child do have any special needs or problems, consult your doctor or a physiotherapist. This book cannot replace medical consultation and should be used in conjunction with professional advice.

contents

Introduction

There is nothing more natural than having a baby, and many parents would tell you that there is no life-experience more rewarding. The sense of achievement that many women feel when they look back on childbirth is unlike any other – even if the birth turned out very differently than they expected, and forty years after the event, most fathers can remember every detail of the moment they saw their child being born.

The birth of your child, however, is just the beginning of the journey of being a parent. Raising a son or daughter is a lifelong project, one that involves, over the course of the years, thousands of separate judgments and decisions that will affect the way your child grows up, and the kind of person he or she becomes. Those decisions, when repeated across the population, also have far-reaching effects on the world at large. For example, there is an ecological price to be paid if everyone, or nearly everyone, exclusively uses disposable nappies (diapers).

This book is intended to help parents to make choices that are soundly natural, responsibly ecological and roundly sensible. Parenting, like any other social activity,

Breastfeeding is the most natural way to feed your new baby, and there is plenty of support out there to help you get the hang of it, and continue.

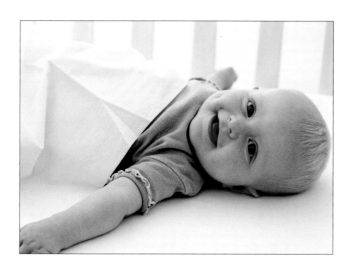

Parents have to make thousands of decisions when they bring up their children. But ultimately the most important thing is that they feel loved and special.

is subject to fashion – but this book is not a trendy guide to green parenthood, and has no ideological axe of its own to grind. The aim of the book is primarily to give parents the means to look after their baby in a way that does as little harm to the environment and the community as possible, but more importantly in a way that is also good for the child.

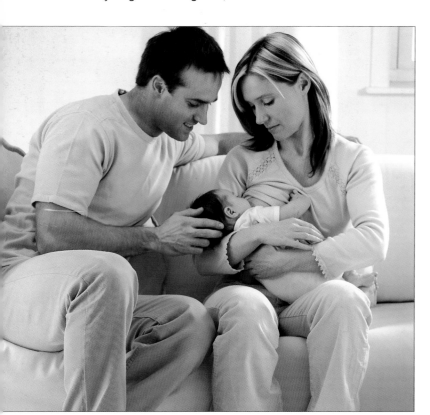

Natural remedies can help you treat some of the common ailments that all children often experience.

Your physical closeness, loving touch and communication are three of the most precious gifts you can give your child.

Children have a natural curiosity about the world, and need the chance to explore it through sight, smell, touch, hearing and taste.

Whenever you can, make daily jobs and tasks a shared activity. Babies and young toddlers can find the most mundane activity entertaining if you are with them.

In practice, natural childcare is an amalgam of old practices (such as breastfeeding rather than using formula, and cooking real food rather than using jars of processed babyfood) and of the best new thinking in paediatrics (such as the revelation that cold, fresh air is the best treatment for croup). There is nothing regressive about using time-honoured methods, nor is it a denial of modern technology. The claim, for example, that breastmilk is the best food for your baby is undeniable; but formula milk and other options are there if you cannot manage it at any point. And the business of using 'real' nappies is much easier in today's society than it was a generation ago: there are washing services, there are

shaped nappies with poppers that are almost as easy to put on as disposables. All these nappy options are better for the world and, crucially in this instance, better for your baby's skin than the bleached, indestructible, chemical-rich disposables that were once seen as a mother's best friend, and the only option readily available.

Any parent who aims to take a natural approach to childcare will find much guidance in these pages – but it is not a manual. The advice given begins with the premise that every parent has an instinctive way of caring for their baby and a growing knowledge of the unique individual their baby is. Trust this instinct, and build on your experience, and you won't go far wrong.

You can protect your child from exposure to many household chemicals by using essential oils and items such as oil and vinegar instead of ordinary cleaners.

When your baby begins to crawl it opens up a whole new world of discovery and independence for them. They will be delighted with their new skill.

section one

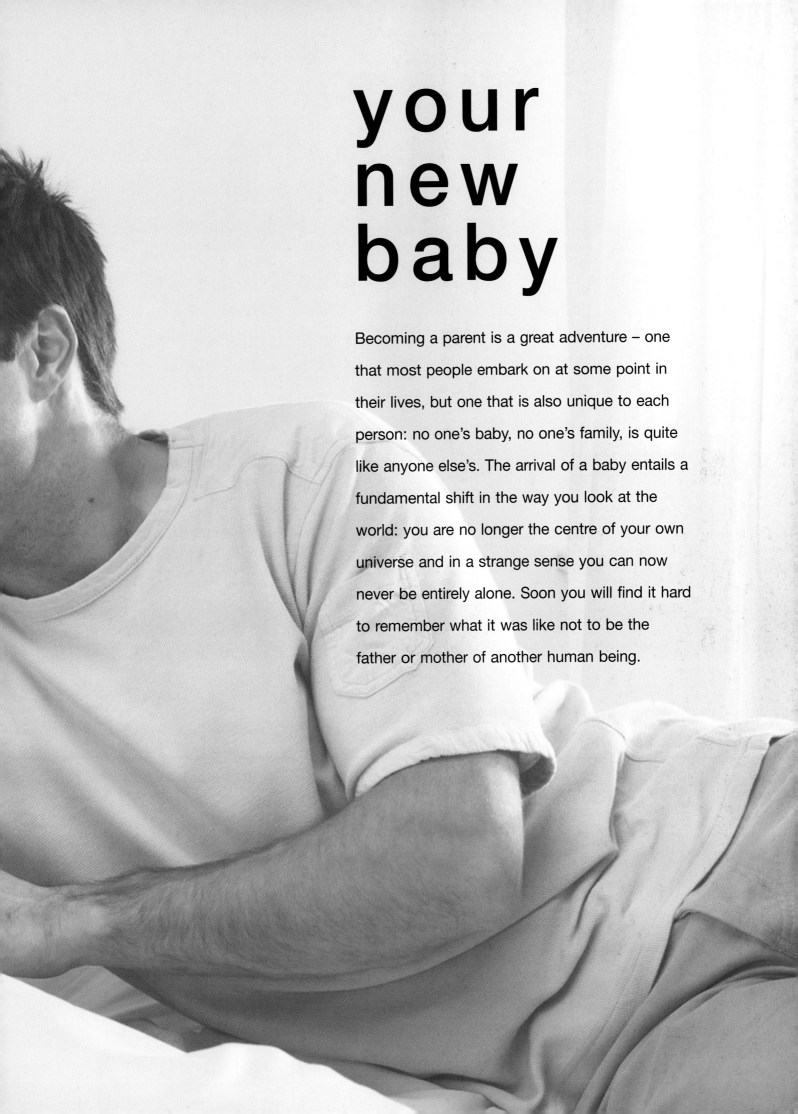

your new baby

Becoming a parent is a great adventure – one that most people embark on at some point in their lives, but one that is also unique to each person: no one's baby, no one's family, is quite like anyone else's. The arrival of a baby entails a fundamental shift in the way you look at the world: you are no longer the centre of your own universe and in a strange sense you can now never be entirely alone. Soon you will find it hard to remember what it was like not to be the father or mother of another human being.

The first days and weeks

" No two babies, not even twins, are the same, and yours will have likes and dislikes right from the start. "

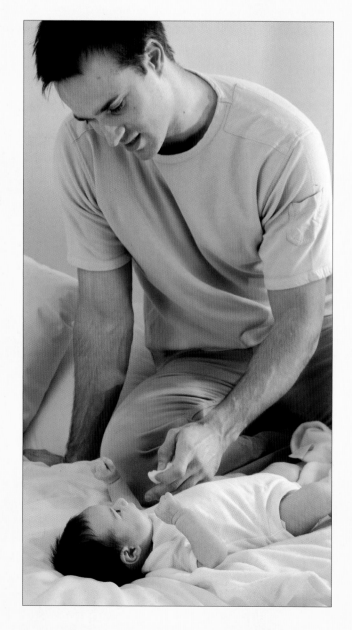

The weeks after a child is born are a time of great transformation for your family. If this is your first baby, you and your partner have stepped over the threshold of parenthood. Here at last is the baby you have been looking forward to for so long. Your life – wonderfully and irreversibly – will never be the same again.

It will help you to enjoy and appreciate this special time if you can give it the importance it deserves. Spend as much time as you can together as a family, limit your visitors to those who will help and support you, and try to let go of other anxieties and concerns – work, money, family problems and so on. Above all, rest and recuperate as much as you can.

There will inevitably be moments – or even long interludes – when you feel you have taken on an almost impossible task. It is entirely normal and extremely common to struggle with fatigue and disorientation at first. You may have feelings of confusion or even despair when, say, your baby is crying and you don't know why. All new parents

The most important thing that a new father can do is to spend time with his baby and partner. Most hospitals will leave the family alone to facilitate bonding.

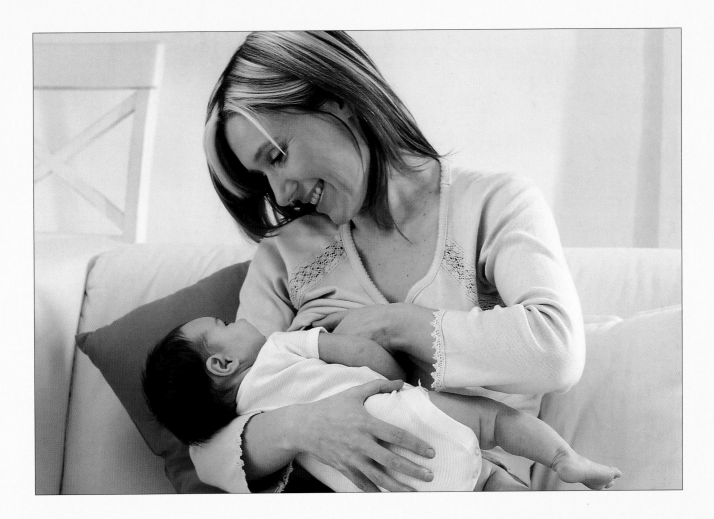

know this experience, and there will come a time when you can look back on the sleepless nights with a rueful smile.

It helps to remember that your child is a unique individual. No two babies, not even twins, are the same, and yours will have likes and dislikes right from the start. You will need to experiment to discover exactly how your baby likes to be held, and whether stroking or patting, for example, soothes him or her more easily. This is much easier if you take a flexible approach, rather than trying to follow a set routine from the outset. Spending these first weeks observing, listening to and cuddling the baby will help you to get to know your child and to understand his or her needs in a way that will store up benefits for the months and years to come.

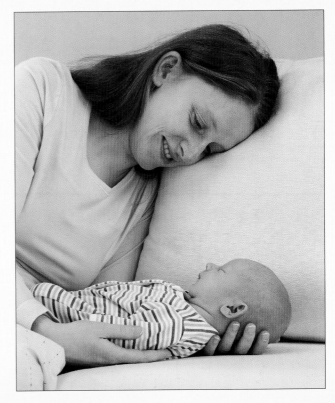

Top: Spend plenty of time getting to know your new baby. An alert baby will be just as curious about you and will gaze upon your face.

Some mothers fall in love with their babies at the first instant, but many women find that they take longer to form a really close attachment.

Bonding with your baby

A lot is said about the importance of bonding straight after the birth, and it is wonderful if the new family can be given the quiet and privacy they need to enjoy these first moments together. Your baby has been propelled from the dark, familiar cocoon of the mother's womb into a bright and noisy world, and is being bombarded with new sensations. In your arms is the most comforting and reassuring place to be.

The hour or so after delivery is also the ideal time to start breastfeeding. It not only encourages bonding but also stimulates digestion and ensures that the baby gets the protective benefits of the first milk (colostrum) straight away. Babies practise the sucking movement while in the womb, and if placed on the mother's stomach may find their own way to the nipple using their sense of smell.

At this time bright lights should be dimmed to create as relaxing and unobtrusive an environment as possible. Any weighing or non-urgent checks should wait, so that mother and baby can get to know each other. The room should be warm so that the baby can be placed naked on the mother's bare skin. If the father is there, he shouldn't feel that he has to immediately rush off to telephone relatives with the news. It is far more important that he stays to share the first few minutes of his baby's life. Everything else can wait.

All babies need loving touch. Research shows that premature babies who are stroked gain more weight, are more responsive and spend fewer days in hospital.

WHEN BONDING IS DELAYED

In the past, mothers and babies in hospital were separated soon after the birth to allow the mother to rest. Fathers' visiting rights were strictly limited. Bonding is now seen as so important that midwives and hospital staff do everything they can to facilitate a new family's need for time alone together. But the safety and health of the baby and mother come first, and if the delivery has been tricky or there are concerns about either, they may have to be separated for a while.

Even if the mother is physically close to her newborn, she may not feel the rush of love that she may have expected. She may be too exhausted from the labour and delivery to be able to feel anything other than relief that it is over; she may be in pain or shock or feeling woozy from the effect of drugs, or she may feel initial disappointment if the child is, say, a boy rather than a girl or has a physical defect such as a hare lip or a birthmark. If she had strong ideas about the type of birth she wanted and it turned out differently, she may be distracted by disappointment and less able to appreciate the beautiful baby in front of her.

Similarly, the father may have found the birth a much more distressing experience than he imagined, especially if there were complications. He may be too worried about his partner to feel much for his child. He may be disturbed

Many new mothers find that they cannot sleep the night after the birth, because they don't want to miss a minute of the child's first hours of life.

to find that the blood-streaked, blotchy newborn that he sees before him does not match the image of the angelic -looking baby he expected. And the realization that he is now responsible for this tiny being may feel overwhelming rather than exciting.

Some parents feel guilty if they do not feel instant love for their baby, and being separated from the child early on can be devastating. But it is a mistake to think that any delay in the bonding process will have a permanent effect on your relationship.

Bonding often starts slowly and grows over time. There is nothing special that you need to do to help this process along. It will unfold naturally as you get to know your baby, as you learn about his or her likes and dislikes, and – especially – as you tend to the baby's needs: changing, cleaning, bathing, comforting, rocking and feeding. Your baby will not remember those first hours of life, but over the months and years that follow will gradually become aware of being encompassed by your love and care.

SPECIAL CARE

Some babies need to be looked after in a special care unit. It can be very hard to see your baby in an incubator or covered in tubes. But even if you cannot yet bring the baby home, there is a lot you can do. Spend as much time as possible by your baby's side, talking softly so that he or she gets to know your voice. Hold the baby's hand and stroke him or her through the holes in the side of the incubator. Cuddle the baby as much you are able: skin-to-skin contact helps to regulate a baby's heartbeat, body temperature and breathing, and it is very calming.

Breastfeeding helps you to bond. It gives you the satisfaction of knowing that you are giving your baby the best possible nourishment and is also the one thing that you can do for your child that nobody else can. If the baby can't be taken out of the incubator, then you can express milk to be given through a tube. The hospital should help you to do this by lending you an efficient breast pump and giving you privacy to use it. It can be hard to establish a good milk supply by expressing alone, so ask for support from a breastfeeding counsellor.

Occasionally a baby needs to be taken to a different hospital for special care while the mother is too ill to travel. This is very distressing, and it will help if the father can become the main carer for a while. If you are a mother in this situation, it is important to remember that you will be able to start the bonding process later on. In the meantime, keep a photograph of your baby with you. Some hospitals use webcams so that parents can see their babies even when they cannot be with them.

Holding a young baby can feel daunting at first. It takes several weeks before new parents feel confident about handling their baby.

Nursing your baby soon after birth gets breastfeeding off to the best possible start. The antibodies in colostrum will help to protect your newborn from infection, and babies who are nursed early on may be less likely to develop sucking problems later.

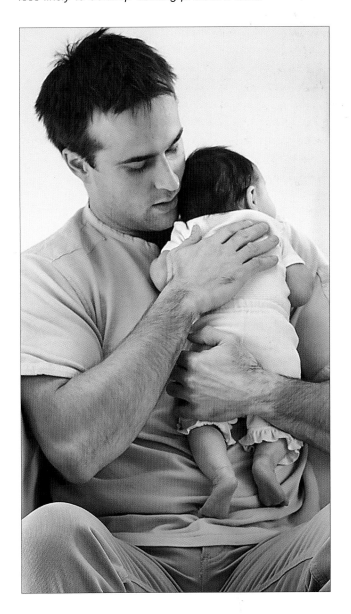

Your newborn baby

Not all newborn babies are cherubic visions of beauty. Their heads may be an odd shape after the birth (especially if the delivery was by ventouse or forceps) and their noses may look squashed. Their eyes may be puffy; their skin (especially if they were overdue) may be wrinkly and flaky, look greasy or be covered in downy hair, and it may have a bluish hue. Their genitals may be slightly swollen. All these strange features are normal and will start to disappear over the next few days and weeks.

WHAT YOUR BABY CAN SENSE

Babies enter the world fully equipped to apprehend and understand their environment. That is, they are in possession of all five senses – sight, hearing, smell, taste and touch – and begin to use them straight away.

Touch. Babies need touch in order to thrive. Your baby is most sensitive to touch around the mouth. Even tiny newborns respond well to gentle stroking, and older babies usually enjoy massage too.

Smell and taste. Research shows that babies have a natural preference for sweet tastes right from the start. They react to smells in the same way as adults: they recoil from bad odours and are drawn to sweet ones. They also quickly learn to differentiate their mother's smell from that of other people.

Hearing. Babies respond to sound in the womb, and may recognize music that they heard regularly before birth. But it is voices that they like best, and they show a preference for their mother's voice above all others. They also show dislike for certain sounds and will jump if they hear a sudden loud noise.

Seeing. Newborns find it easiest to focus on objects 20–30cm/8–12in away – roughly the distance of your face when you hold a baby in your arms or breastfeed. Babies show the most interest in faces, but are also fascinated by simple patterns.

Babies don't have the muscle power to hold up their heavy heads, so you must keep a newborn's head well supported at all times. Gradually, the muscles in the neck grow stronger and they will be able to support the head, but watch out for sudden lapses as the head lolls.

YOUR BABY'S REFLEXES

A newborn baby is entirely dependent on your care, but is born with some instinctive reactions designed to help him or her survive.

Rooting, sucking and swallowing: If stroked on the cheek, a baby will turn and search for the nipple (this is called rooting). Babies suck when they feel pressure on the hard palate in the mouth, and swallow automatically.

Gripping. If you put a finger in your baby's hand, he or she will grasp it. Your baby will also curl the feet if the soles are touched. These reflexes are left over from our primate ancestors, who needed to cling to their mothers' fur. They gradually develop into a deliberate holding action.

Crawling. When placed on their tummies, babies will curl their legs and arms beneath their bodies and may even produce a crawl-like movement. Gradually your baby's body uncurls from its foetal position and he or she will lie flat.

Stepping. If they are held so that their feet touch a firm surface, newborn babies will lift one foot after another in a stepping motion. This reflex disappears after a few days, and has to be re-learnt many months later when it is time to learn to walk.

Startle reflex. If newborns are startled, they fling out their arms and legs as if to grab hold of something. Your baby finds this distressing, so see it as a reminder that he or she should be handled gently. The reflex disappears at about two months.

Lifting and putting down your baby

Babies need to be held securely and comfortably in the first few weeks, until their neck muscles have developed enough for them to support their own head. Always lift your baby slowly and gently to avoid startling him or her.

1 Alert the baby to your presence first by speaking softly, and putting your hand on their tummy. Lean over so that your body is close to the baby, and slide one hand under the head and neck.

2 Slide the other hand under the lower back and bottom. Take the baby's weight into your hands, and then bring him or her slowly towards you. When your baby is resting on your chest, begin to sit upright.

3 When putting the baby down, hold him or her close to you as you bend over. This means that the baby doesn't have to travel too far in mid-air. Keep your hands in position for a while before sliding them out.

HOW YOUR BABY COMMUNICATES

As helpless as newborns are, they can communicate in a way that almost guarantees they get their basic needs met: they cry. At first your baby's cries will all sound the same to you. But in time you may notice that he or she makes different sounds depending on what is wrong, and you may learn to distinguish between, say, a cry that means "I'm hungry" and one that says "I'm in pain". After a few weeks, your baby will also start to communicate pleasure, by gurgling, cooing and making other repetitive little noises.

The person who looks after the baby most often – usually a parent – will probably see the first smile, which comes by about six weeks. At first babies will smile at any face – including a picture of one – by three months they smile more readily at the people they know best.

THE FONTANELLE

The bones of a newborn's skull have not yet fused together. The gaps between the bones, called fontanelles, are covered by a tough membrane and can't be damaged by normal handling. The largest one is on the crown of the baby's head, you may be able to see a pulse beating through it. This fontanelle can indicate a baby's state of health. If it is sunken, the baby is dehydrated and needs fluids urgently. A bulging fontanelle is another sign of illness, which also needs immediate medical attention.

Carrying your baby

When carrying your baby, both of you need to feel confident and secure. There are two safe ways to hold your newborn baby: the shoulder hold, which is good for winding and for general carrying around, and the cradle hold, which is a soothing way to nurse your baby.

1 For the shoulder hold, support the baby against your chest, so that his or her head leans against your shoulder. Use one hand to support the bottom and back, and keep the other behind the back and head to stop the baby jerking backwards.

2 To use the cradle hold, hold the baby by resting his or her head and shoulders in the crook of your arm, and use your other hand to support the bottom and lower back. Newborn babies will feel most safe and secure held closely against your body.

The first weeks

In many cultures, it is traditional for the mother to stay indoors for 40 days after the birth – one for each week of pregnancy. During this time she is released from the burden of household chores, given special foods to restore her strength and encouraged to stay in bed to bond with her infant. Bedouin Arabs, Jews, Somalis and Latin Americans all observe 40 days of seclusion, while Chinese women "do the month".

Until very recently, western women were also encouraged to rest after giving birth – your grandmother probably spent a week or two "lying-in", either in hospital or at home. But today new mothers are under immense pressure to get back to normal, regain their figures and show the baby off to all their relatives. This makes the first weeks after childbirth more exhausting and stressful than they need to be.

When you are caring for a small baby it is easy to forget to drink enough. Have a jug or bottle of water to hand.

RESTORATIVE TEA

A spicy hot drink can invigorate and energize you. This mixture includes raspberry leaf tea, which encourages the healthy contraction of the womb, and nettle tea, which is a traditional tonic. Drink up to three cups a day.

3 cardamon pods
3 cloves
5cm/2in stick of cinnamon
2.5cm/1in chunk of ginger, sliced
3 tsp raspberry leaf tea
3 tsp nettle tea

Put 750ml/30fl oz water in a small, lidded pan and add the spices. Bring to the boil, cover and simmer for 10 minutes. Add the teas to the spice mixture, steep for 10 minutes then strain into a flask to keep warm. Drink when required.

A MODERN LYING-IN

It makes sense to withdraw from society for a while so that you can concentrate on your new baby. Everyone's idea of lying-in will be different, but it can be helpful to do the following, at least for a week or two.

Stay at home and don't get dressed. Pyjamas or a nightie are much more comfortable to wear than day clothes, and they help to remind you (and any visitors) that you are resting.

Make your bedroom the centre of your existence. Have everything you need close at hand – water, a bowl of fruit, healthy snacks, phone, books or magazines – to make this time pleasurable.

A new baby is happiest cuddled close against the breast. If the contact is skin to skin, even better, as your scent will add to the feeling of security.

If you are going to be on your own at home with a new baby, make sure you have plenty of healthy food that is quick to prepare and easy to eat.

Fathers will also need to get rest whenever they can. It is tempting to fall asleep together on the sofa, but don't, as the baby could become trapped between cushions.

Keep your baby with you all or most of the time. Follow his or her rhythms – feed the baby on demand, sleep when he or she sleeps.

Have another adult around. Ideally, the father will be at home to look after you and share the care of the baby. But if that isn't possible, ask your mother, best friend or another person close to you to stay.

Eat well. Have at least one hot meal a day (cooked by someone else) and lots of healthy, easy-to-prepare snacks at other times – fruit, cereal, yoghurt, oatcakes, smoked salmon, cold meats and so on. Make sure you drink lots of water.

Limit first visitors to close friends and family. For the first few weeks, arrange visits at times that are convenient to you, and keep them short. Ask your partner or supporter to encourage people gently to leave if you start to get tired.

If people offer help, accept it. Ask them to bring you a cooked meal or do some housework, so that you and your partner can concentrate on the baby.

Keep your first outings short and pleasurable. It is quite normal to feel a little strange at first. Many traditional cultures have a celebration at the end of the seclusion period, which serves not only to welcome the new baby but also to help reintegrate the mother into the world.

LOVING CARE FOR YOUR BABY

Looking after a newborn can feel daunting, not least because new parents are inundated with advice. Do ignore suggestions from well-meaning friends and relatives if they don't feel right for you at this moment.

What works for one baby doesn't necessarily work for another, and women who had their babies years ago – including your own mother and mother-in-law – may have ideas that are out of date.

The most important thing is to spend lots of relaxed time with your baby, concentrating completely on him or her, with no distractions, so that you get to know each other. Gradually, you will discover how to tell when the baby is hungry or tired, how he or she likes to be carried and what is most soothing, being rocked or shushed for example. This takes time, and it is important to trust your own instincts as you learn. In the meantime, the following pointers may help.

Babies thrive on physical contact. Cuddle your baby as much as you can, and limit the amount of time spent in a bouncy chair or pram.

Prioritize breastfeeding. As well as meeting your baby's basic needs for food and drink, it brings you physically close and helps with bonding.

Don't spend longer than an hour or two away from your baby. It's natural for mothers to want to be near their newborns, but other people can confuse you by telling you that you need time to yourself, and grandparents in particular may push to "have a turn" at looking after the baby. Don't worry about other people's needs just now, and give in to this kind of pressure only if you really feel that you need a break.

The father is important, too. For the first year or so, the mother is usually at the centre of her baby's world, but the father will develop a much closer relationship with his child if he is involved in day-to-day care: changing nappies (diapers), cleaning, bathing and comforting. Fathers are often better than mothers at soothing babies who are distressed or windy, because the babies pick up on their mothers' anxiety.

Common problems for infants

Even the most beautiful and natural of births is physically gruelling for the baby, who is pushed and squeezed down the narrow birth canal. So it is not surprising that newborns are often bruised and marked and sometimes have bloodshot eyes. These little blemishes will fade in a few days and need no treatment.

If you have had a forceps or ventouse delivery, the baby's head may be misshapen for a while. This too will correct itself naturally. However, a baby who has had an assisted delivery may have a headache for a few days, which can make him or her cry more than normal. Lots of cuddling and nursing will help. If your baby continues to be very fractious, then gentle massage can help. It may also be worth taking the baby to a cranial osteopath, who can gently correct any distortions in the skull.

BIRTHMARKS
Some babies are born with a birthmark that is permanent. Three in every thousand have a pink or purple port-wine stain. This often occurs on the face, and is very occasionally linked to problems such as epilepsy. It can be upsetting when your child has a birthmark of this nature, and it may take time for their parents to come to terms with it. However, port-wine stains can be treated with lasers which can radically improve their appearance. Very occasionally, a baby is born with a raised brown mole. It's important to keep an eye on this and seek medical advice if it changes colour, shape or size: a mole can be surgically removed if there is cause for concern.

Breastmilk has natural antibacterial properties, so it is the perfect cleanser for a newborn's sticky eye.

It is thought that stork marks may be the result of pressure on the head once the baby engages.

Strawberry marks can be quite prominent, but they usually fade and then disappear in a few years.

TEMPORARY BIRTHMARKS, SPOTS AND RASHES
Stork marks are so-called because it is fancifully said that they are caused by the beak of the mythical stork that delivers babies. They are pink or red marks on the brow, eyelids or back of the neck, which become more prominent when the baby cries. They gradually fade but can take up to two years to disappear completely.

Strawberry marks are red marks that start off flat and gradually become raised, increasing in size. They can be present at birth or develop a few days later. They have usually gone by the time the child is two or three. Mongolian spots are blue or grey patches that can appear on the buttocks or back. They affect black or Asian babies, and usually disappear by the end of the first year.

Most newborn babies develop minor skin problems in their first weeks. Heat rashes (tiny red spots) are very common because babies have immature sweat glands and are unable to control their temperature efficiently. If

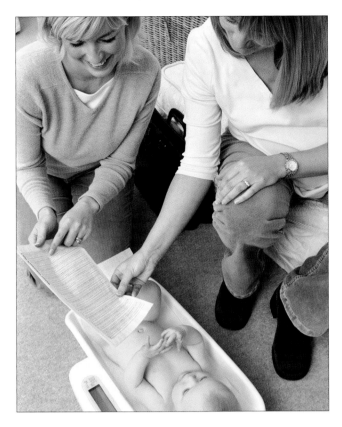

Babies may be weighed often in the early weeks to see that they are growing normally. Frequent checking can feel rather stressful for the parents, but so long as the overall weight gain is steady and your baby looks fit and healthy, there is nothing to worry about.

the sweat glands become blocked, tiny white spots (milia or milk spots) appear. They will disappear of their own accord in a few weeks. Do not pick at them or you may cause infection.

STICKY EYE

The eyes of newborns can produce a sticky, yellowish discharge. If this occurs in the first day or two it usually means they have picked up an infection in the birth canal. Use a cotton-wool pad (cotton ball) soaked in cooled, boiled water, or breast milk, to clean each eye, wiping from the nose outwards. See a doctor if it persists.

JAUNDICE

More than half of newborn babies develop jaundice two or three days after the birth. This is not a disease but a symptom: it means that bilirubin (a pigment produced by the body when red blood cells are broken down) has built up in their system. Usually the liver processes bilirubin, but a baby's immature liver is unable to cope with all the extra bilirubin produced when large amounts of red blood cells are broken down after the birth.

In most cases, the signs of jaundice are a yellowing of the whites of the eyes and the skin (which usually starts on the head and spreads down the chest and stomach).

Your midwife should check for jaundice but do point it out if you are concerned. Usually, no treatment is needed, and the jaundice clears up in a week or two. (In premature babies, who develop it five to seven days after the birth, it can take up to two months to disappear.)

If your baby's jaundice reaches the arms and legs, or there are other symptoms such as difficulty sucking, sleepiness, dark urine or pale stools, see your doctor promptly. Occasionally jaundice can have a serious cause, such as liver problems. The usual treatment is light therapy (phototherapy), which is done in hospital, but very occasionally a blood transfusion is needed.

INFECTED UMBILICAL CORD

It can take up to four weeks for the stump of the baby's umbilical cord to shrink and drop off, leaving a small wound that will heal in a few days. Doctors sometimes advise dabbing the stump with rubbing alcohol to prevent infection, but recent research suggests that it is best left to dry by itself. Clean the area around the stump daily with cooled, boiled water and pat dry with a clean towel. Fold down the top of the nappy so that air can reach the area. This will help it to heal faster. If the stump starts to ooze pus or smell, or the surrounding area becomes red, see a doctor, who will prescribe antibiotic cream.

THE SIX-WEEK CHECK

Babies are checked from head to toe soon after the birth and again six weeks later. At the six-week check, you'll be asked about your baby's feeding and sleeping patterns, as well as what you have noticed about his or her hearing and vision. The baby will be weighed (naked) and measured, and the results plotted on a centile chart to see how he or she compares with the national averages. The baby's vision, head control and muscle tone will be systematically checked and a hearing test may be done. The doctor will also look at your baby's eyes, heart, spine, hips and genitals to ensure all is well.

Common problems for new mothers

Every woman needs time to recover from giving birth. Even if you have had a natural vaginal delivery with no tearing, you are likely to feel bruised and tired. You may have aches and pains in odd places, especially if you had an active birth in which you moved around a lot. And, of course, your body is adjusting to the fact that you are no longer pregnant: your womb is shrinking back to its normal size, your hormone levels have dropped and your breasts are producing milk to sustain your new baby.

Much of the discomfort experienced by new mothers can be eased with the help of natural remedies. None of the remedies given will interfere with breastfeeding. However, it is important to see your doctor or midwife if you have severe pain or are worried about any symptom.

Afterpains are often at their most intense when you are breastfeeding, because this triggers the release of the hormone oxytocin, which encourages the womb to contract. Sit in a relaxed position and breathe slowly and deeply and relax your muscles to ease the cramp.

AFTERPAINS

Many women experience cramp-like pains in the abdomen when the womb starts to contract. These start within hours of the birth and usually last three days at most (often less). Afterpains can be intense, particularly during breastfeeding. They also tend to be stronger with second and subsequent children, as the womb becomes increasingly stretched.

There are simple things you can do to ease the discomfort: a warm bath or a warm hot-water bottle held against the abdomen help to relax the muscles. Sipping a soothing herbal tea such as chamomile, or an antispasmodic one such as ginger or crampbark, may also help. Raspberry leaf tea, so useful for strengthening the womb before childbirth, also helps it to readjust afterwards. Some women swear by the homeopathic remedy Mag phos, and Chamomilla can also be helpful.

SORE PERINEUM

If you have had a natural birth, your perineal area will have been stretched, so it will feel sore and bruised. Homeopathic Arnica tablets are excellent for treating the bruising, and will also help with any shock resulting from the birth. Doing your pelvic floor exercises will speed healing, since these encourage blood to flow to the area.

Take one or two warm baths a day to encourage healing and give you a few precious minutes to yourself; dilute a few drops each of tea tree and lavender oil in a carrier oil and add to the water. For immediate relief, apply a pad of cotton wool (cotton ball) soaked in witch hazel. Alternatively, use a home-made icepack (made by wrapping ice in a plastic bag then covering it in two layers of kitchen paper or a cotton cloth), but don't use this for longer than ten minutes at a time.

As you urinate, pour a jug of lukewarm water over the perineal area to prevent stinging. Pat rather than wipe it

Include plenty of fresh vegetables and wholegrain cereals, including oats and bran, in your diet before and after childbirth to ensure that you get enough fibre and help prevent constipation.

Lavender and tea tree oils can help the healing of tears or cuts. Add 2–3 drops to a warm bath.

An ice pack – applied for up to ten minutes – can bring welcome relief to a bruised perineum.

dry. Many women worry about how it will feel when they move their bowels for the first time. You may be concerned that your stitches will tear, but be assured that they won't. However, the first bowel movements after childbirth will be more difficult if you are constipated, so drink plenty of fluids and eat lots of fruits and vegetables.

HAEMORRHOIDS

Even if you got through pregnancy without developing haemorrhoids, also called piles, they may well develop when you are pushing down in labour (about one-third of women get them after a vaginal delivery). If you don't have any itching or pain, you can leave them to heal naturally, but taking warm baths and doing pelvic floor exercises will be helpful.

The homeopathic remedy Hamamelis is often recommended for itchy or painful piles. You can apply a pad soaked in witch hazel to the area: this is cooling and

The homeopathic remedy Chamomilla can help with afterpains. You could also try sipping a cup of chamomile tea three times a day.

encourages shrinking. You can smooth Calendula cream on the piles between compresses. It's important to avoid becoming constipated (see above), since this will exacerbate the problem. Wash the area with water and pat dry after each bowel movement.

AFTER A CAESAREAN

If you had your baby by Caesarean section, recovery will take a little longer than with a natural birth – you have had major abdominal surgery, after all. You'll be encouraged to get moving as soon as possible in order to start the healing process, and you may be given gentle exercises to practise. But you will have to be careful about how you move and should avoid lifting anything heavier than your baby for at least six weeks. You should not drive for at least a month. Check this with your insurance company.

It is important to keep the Caesarean scar clean and dry. Frequent baths will help with healing; adding lavender and tea tree essential oils may prevent infection. Carefully pat the area dry afterwards, or use a hairdryer on a low setting. Arnica tablets are good for bruising and shock. Once the scar has healed, you can massage it daily with lavender oil and vitamin E oil diluted in a blend of almond and wheatgerm carrier oils.

THE POSTNATAL CHECK

All new mothers are invited to a check-up with their doctor about six weeks after the birth. This is usually done in tandem with the baby's six-week check. You'll be asked about how you are recovering and the doctor will examine you to see if any tears have healed. This is a good time to voice any concerns you have about any aspect of your recovery.

Handling your emotions

Giving birth is an incredible experience, often the most powerfully emotional event of a woman's life. But there is little time for you to reflect on it because there is a tiny, vulnerable baby needing round-the-clock care. Not surprisingly, the first few days after the birth can be a very emotional and bewildering time for both parents. You may feel exhilarated and joyous, exhausted and overwhelmed, proud and fearful, often in quick succession.

As a new mother, it is helpful to remember that your hormones are out of balance, and the physical opening of the body for childbirth has affected you on a deep emotional level. In a way, it would be odd if you felt utterly serene and completely in control as you adjust to the new person in your life.

BABY BLUES
About half of all new mothers get very tearful or anxious a few days after the baby is born, and it is common to experience mood swings. These "baby blues" are probably due to the sharp drop in hormone levels, and they may also be connected with feelings of anticlimax after the intensity of the birth. The most helpful way of dealing with them is to relax, and allow yourself to feel the emotions. Cry if you need to, and be open about how you are feeling to your partner or to a good friend.

A healthy diet, with red meat for iron and oily fish for essential fatty acids, can help you to manage difficult emotions after the birth, and helps breastfeeding too.

EMOTIONAL STRENGTH PLAN
The baby blues are usually temporary, but can sometimes come and go over a few weeks. Prioritize your physical needs – eat healthily and often so that your blood-sugar levels don't drop, drink plenty of fluid and sleep whenever your baby does.

Good nutrition can help with depression. The fatty acids in oily fish help maintain a healthy nervous system; calcium (found in dairy products, green vegetables, nuts and seeds, beans and lentils) and magnesium (nuts and seeds, green leafy vegetables, wheatgerm, sprouted grains, soy beans and whole grains) are also helpful. Check your iron levels – anaemia makes you feel lethargic and one study found that low iron levels could hamper bonding. Liquid iron is more easily digested than tablets, while good nutritional sources are lean red meat, oily fish, pulses, nuts, dark green vegetables and dried fruit. Vitamin C helps your body to absorb iron: citrus fruits are a good source. In addition, doing the following will help keep you in good emotional health and will help you to get through any periods of unhappiness or low spirits.
- Be open about how you are feeling with your partner, close friends and health professionals.
- Talk to your midwife about the birth experience. This can be very useful if you have any ambivalent feelings about your labour or delivery.
- Treat yourself to a postnatal massage or acupuncture treatment. Some complementary therapists will come to your home.

Rescue Remedy is a good instant remedy for any feelings of anxiety, panic or fearfulness.

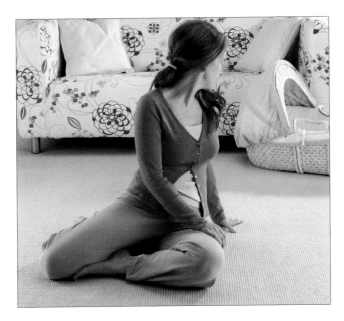

Yoga, or gentle stretching exercises, can have a calming effect and may help to counter feelings of depression.

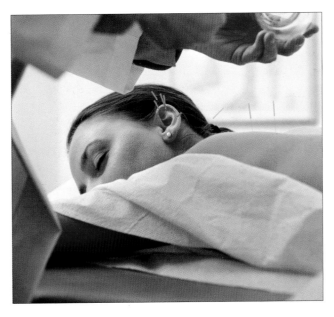

An acupuncture treatment can help you to feel more balanced after the exertion of giving birth.

- If you are on your own with the baby, make sure you see somebody every day. If you feel low, do some physical exercise every day, such as brisk walking and postnatal yoga. After six weeks – provided you get the all clear from your doctor – try a gentle postnatal circuit class or go swimming.

POSTNATAL DEPRESSION

Quite different to the baby blues, postnatal depression (PND) can start weeks or months after the birth, and can be long-lasting. It can make a woman feel so exhausted and lethargic that looking after the baby feels an impossible task, and it may cause anxiety and strong feelings of inadequacy. Fathers can also sometimes suffer from depression after the birth of a child.

Depression is hard to diagnose because it is normal to feel low and inadequate from time to time, but if feelings like this persist for more than a week or so you should seek medical help. There are various treatments for postnatal depression. Practical help, counselling, support groups and, if necessary, medication can all be helpful.

FIRST DAYS AS A DAD

It can be hard to be a new father. You are the parent of a tiny baby, which can feel overwhelming. Your relationship with your partner is likely to feel very different for a while and you may feel excluded by the bond between mother and child, especially if the baby is being breastfed. As new mothers tend to be tired and hormonal, your partner may seem irritable and unappreciative at first. The thrill of fatherhood is no less real or satisfying than the joy of

A new father may feel thrilled with his tiny child, but have moments of feeling overwhelmed or panicked too.

motherhood, however, and most fathers quickly carve out a role that is all their own, such as taking charge of bathtime or the first change of the day. Such things – however mundane they seem at the time – lay the foundation for the special and unique relationship between a man and his child.

Once the initial month or two are past, you will find that the presence of your child adds a whole new dimension to your relationship with your partner. Your baby is, after all, a tangible and constant sign of your love, a wonderful lifelong link between you.

Basic baby care and feeding

> 66 Breastfeeding naturally binds mother and baby together, making them inseparable for the first months of a child's life. 99

Lots of people talk about the hard work involved in looking after a baby. And it is true that a small baby requires almost constant care and attention. But there is also great pleasure to be had from lovingly attending to your child's needs.

These needs are, generally, pretty straightforward. Babies want feeding, probably more often and more erratically than you can imagine; they need changing when they are wet or dirty; they need to be kept warm; and they need to be held so that they feel safe. All these things are easily done, but the way you go about them can make all the difference between enjoying caring for your baby and finding it a burden or chore.

For instance, changing a nappy (certainly one of the less pleasant aspects of parenthood) is much more than a messy cleaning task. It is, in a strange way, a means of communicating your feelings towards your baby. When you put a towel on the cold changing mat to make it more comfortable, or speak soothingly as you touch and clean your baby, you are

A new arrival brings change and excitement to the wider family, as well as the parents. Siblings will want to be involved in caring for the new member of the family.

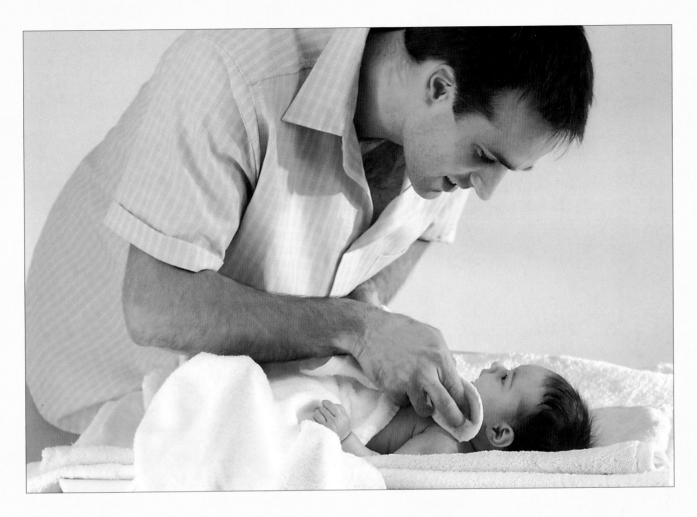

working to make the experience a positive one. Such attentiveness both requires and builds the loving tenderness a parent feels for his or her child.

Nature, through breastfeeding, has provided women with the perfect way to nurture their babies. Breastfeeding naturally binds mother and baby together, making them inseparable for the first months of a child's life. And while this might mean that as a new mother you cannot go out as you used to, it gives you the most wonderful opportunity to give yourself up to motherhood and to forge an unbreakable emotional connection with your child. If you decide to bottle-feed, you can make that connection in the same way, so long as you make a conscious decision to treat feeds as a special time to love and bond with, as well as nourish, your baby.

Top: Looking after a baby involves doing lots of small and repetitive tasks – but these can be incredibly fulfilling and enjoyable.

A baby's father will be able to find lots of ways to care for, and bond with, his child, even a breastfed one. Spend as much time as you can with each other.

Changing your baby

It's worth thinking about what type of nappy (diaper) you are going to use for your new baby before you give birth, so you can plan ahead. Parents spend a lot of time changing nappies. Your baby may need anything up to 12 a day at first, and could easily go through 4,000 nappies in the first two years. You should change your baby immediately a nappy is soiled, and at least every three hours otherwise. However, don't wake your baby up just for a nappy change.

WHICH NAPPY?

You can choose between disposable or cloth nappies, or you can use a combination of both. Disposables are convenient and quick to put on, but it's worth considering cloth nappies, especially if you are trying to reduce the amount of waste your family produces. Real nappies are better for babies' skin than disposables because they are

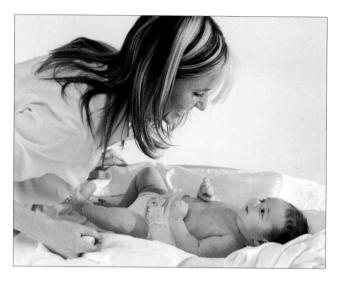

Smiles, eye contact and chat will help your baby to put up with having his or her nappy changed.

REUSEABLE NAPPIES

If you plan to use cloth nappies all the time, you'll need about 24 nappies and three covers. But if you plan to use some disposables, 10 cloth nappies and two waterproof covers should be sufficient. You'll also need two or three booster pads for nighttime, as well as liners. You can get flushable paper liners or reusable cloth or fleece ones.

Terry squares. These are the traditional option and the cheapest. They are good for newborns – a shaped nappy can look huge on a tiny baby. You can now buy plastic fasteners, which are safer than traditional pins.

Prefolds. These nappies are rectangular and have to be folded before use. They come in different sizes, so you will have to buy new ones as the baby grows, but prefolds are generally less expensive than shaped or all-in-one nappies.

Tie-up nappies. These come in one size and are folded in different ways depending on the size of your baby. They are secured using the attached ties.

Shaped nappies. These are probably the easiest to use, because they don't need folding. They come in a range of sizes, or in one size fastened differently depending on the size of the baby, and are secured by poppers or Velcro.

All-in-ones. These are shaped nappies that incorporate a waterproof cover. They are quick to put on, but they take longer to dry after washing and are also more expensive than other nappies. But they can be a good option for when you are out for the day, if you prefer never to use disposables.

shaped nappy

all-in-one

terry squares

plastic fasteners

prefold nappy

tie-up nappy

Nappy fold for a newborn

Even if you intend to use shaped nappies, it is worth investing in some terries for when your baby is very small.

As with other forms of real nappies, you'll need a waterproof liner to prevent leakage.

1 Fold the square in half lengthwise to make a rectangle, then again to make a small square.

2 With the four corners of the nappy at the top, pull the corner of the top layer across to make a triangle.

3 Turn the nappy over and fold the square edge over twice, so it forms a pad in the middle of the triangle.

4 Add a liner, put the baby on the nappy, fold up the base, bring one side over the other and secure .

Kite fold

The newborn fold is good for the first few weeks, but your baby will soon be too big for nappies folded in this way.

The kite fold is suitable for larger babies, and will extend the length of time you can use terry squares.

1 Place the square so that one corner is pointing towards you. Fold in the two side corners to make a basic kite shape.

2 Fold down the pointed top, then fold up the point at the bottom, as shown.

3 Place the baby on the nappy so that his or her waist is aligned with the top edge of the nappy.

4 Fold up the base, then fold one side over the other and secure with a nappy pin or plastic fastener.

made of natural fabrics and don't contain adhesives or superabsorbant chemicals, which can come into contact with the baby's skin. In the long term, real nappies work out cheaper than disposables, especially since you can re-use them for any other children you have. A local nappy laundering service, which delivers clean nappies and collects your dirty ones, is an alternative costing about the same in the end as using disposables.

If you prefer to use disposable nappies, consider using the eco-friendly brands that are now available from health stores, by mail order, on the internet and in some supermarkets. These have fewer chemicals and bleaching agents than most disposables, and contain more biodegradable materials. However, they tend to be more expensive – and bulkier – than ordinary disposables.

WASHING NAPPIES

You will need a large bucket with a tight-fitting lid to store used nappies, until you have enough to make up a wash that fills the machine. If you want to soak the nappies before washing (it isn't essential), add a few drops of tea tree oil – which has antiseptic qualities – or lavender oil to reduce smells, to the water.

To help keep the nappies free from stains, you can also add a tablespoon of bicarbonate of soda or two tablespoons of white vinegar. It is worth buying a mesh bag for the bucket to make it easier to get the nappies into the washing machine: when you are ready to wash, you simply transfer the whole bag to the machine. Use non-biological detergent, and close any Velcro fasteners to prevent snagging.

CHANGING YOUR BABY

During the day, make nappy changing fun. This is a great time for play – talk and sing to your baby, blow raspberries on his or her tummy, make silly expressions to make the baby laugh. Hang a mobile or mirror above your

Change your baby on a changing station or bed to ease your back and knees. Get everything to hand before you begin, and don't leave the baby alone for a second if the mat is above floor level.

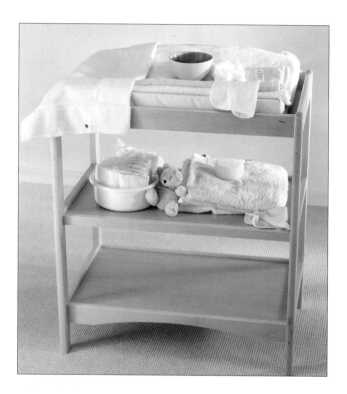

changing area as a distraction. At night, on the other hand, change your baby only if he or she is very wet or has soiled a nappy. Keep the room quiet and dim so that you don't disturb the baby any more than necessary.

CLEARING UP

Put disposable nappies in a nappy sack – you can get biodegradable ones that are made from starch rather than plastic. If you are using cloth nappies, flush soiled paper liners down the toilet and put wet ones in a nappy sack. Hold a soiled reusable liner in the toilet while you flush to rinse it, then place with the nappy in your nappy bucket. Wash your hands with soap and hot water.

PREVENTING AND TREATING NAPPY RASH

Most babies get nappy rash at some point. The best way to prevent it is by keeping your baby clean and dry: he or she is much less likely to get a rash if changed eight times a day or more, and if you leave the nappy off from time to time. It will also help if you use only damp cotton wool to clean the skin, and avoid wipes (especially those that contain alcohol), soap and strong detergents.

If your baby develops any redness, change him or her more often, and leave the nappy off for a few minutes at every change to let air circulate – give longer periods of

CAUTION
Don't use talcum powder on babies: they can inhale the tiny particles, which may be harmful to the lungs.

Cleaning and changing

Get everything ready before you start and have it close to hand. Cover the changing mat with a towel to make it more comfortable and to soak up any accidents. Keep talking to your baby to reassure him or her.

1 Remove lower clothing, and unfasten the nappy. If the stools are very liquid, use some tissue to clean off the worst of it, then clean the baby's bottom using wet cotton wool balls (cotton balls).

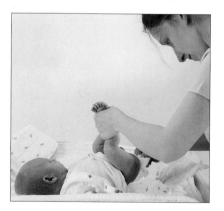

2 Lift up the baby's legs, fold the nappy in half and remove. Clean thoroughly, including creases in the legs. Wipe a girl from front to back. Clean under a boy's testicles but don't pull back the foreskin.

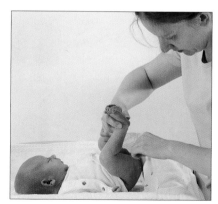

3 if there is any redness, apply a thin smear of barrier cream. Lift the baby by the ankles, then lay the clean nappy underneath, aligning the top of the back with the baby's waist. Lower the baby on to it and fasten it.

There are lots of nappy wipes on the market, but it is best to use cotton wool (cotton balls) and cooled, boiled water to clean your baby, especially in the first weeks. If you need to use wipes when away from home, use unbleached, chemical-free ones.

bare-bottom time if you can. Use a natural barrier cream, such as calendula nappy rash cream, at every change. See your doctor if the rash doesn't clear up within a few days or if blisters or pimples develop.

A GUIDE TO STOOLS

Babies' vary enormously in the number of soiled nappies they produce. Many will move their bowels at every feed, while some breastfed babies can go for up to a week without having a bowel movement. So long as the stools are normal and your baby is not in discomfort, this is nothing to worry about.

Normal stools. A baby's first bowel movement is black or green and very sticky: this is called meconium and it is passed in the first couple of days after the birth. Subsequent stools are usually yellowish in colour. In breastfed babies, they can be mustard yellow and runny

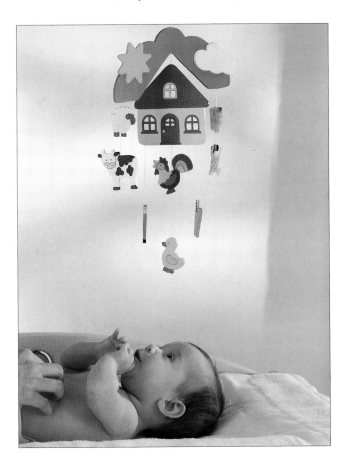

NATURAL SPRAY CLEANER
Bacteria can breed on a changing mat so make sure that you keep it clean. To make your own natural antibacterial cleaner, put two cups of cooled, boiled water in a new, washed, plant-spray bottle. Add 15 drops each of tea tree and mandarin essential oils and shake well before using.

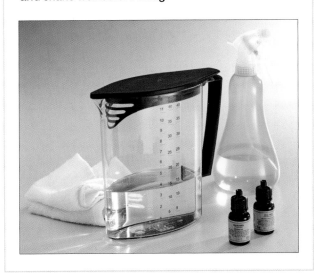

or dark yellow/light brown and grainy. The stools of bottle-fed babies tend to be dark yellow to light brown and firmer than those of breastfed babies.

Green stools. Some formulas can make a baby's stools green, but if they are also slimy, foul-smelling and frequent, then your baby probably has diarrhoea and should be checked by a doctor. A bottle-fed baby may need to drink cooled boiled water instead of formula for a short period; a breastfed baby can feed as normal. A breastfed baby may produce green, watery stools if he or she is getting too much foremilk and not enough of the rich hindmilk. To correct this, make sure the baby has emptied one breast before starting on the other.

Pellet-like brown stools. These suggest constipation. Breastfed babies almost never become constipated because breastmilk is easily digested, but bottle-fed babies may have this problem from time to time. Give cooled boiled water to drink as well as milk and make sure that you are using the correct amount of formula when making up the bottles.

Abnormal stools. Dark brown or black stools (other than meconium) in a young baby may indicate bleeding in the bowel: see your doctor for advice as soon as possible. Dark red or bloody stools may indicate an obstruction in the bowel, this must be checked urgently. Very pale stools may be a sign of jaundice and also must be checked with your doctor.

Hang a colourful mobile above your changing station so that your baby has something to look at.

Bathing your baby

Until a few years ago, mothers were taught how to bath their babies while still in hospital and a bath was seen as an essential part of the daily routine. However, frequent baths are not only unnecessary but also dry out a baby's skin. They can also be upsetting for young babies, who often don't like being naked, and stressful for parents. Handling a slippery infant with a floppy neck can be difficult, especially if he or she is screaming in protest. If your baby screams when you put him or her in the bath, wait a few days and then try again.

If you can, wait two to four weeks before giving the first bath. You can easily keep the baby clean in the meantime by washing his or her bottom at each nappy change, and topping and tailing at least once a day.

NAIL CARE

Most parents find the idea of cutting their baby's tiny nails daunting, but there is no avoiding it. Scratch mittens are useful for the first days, but you can't keep your baby's hands hidden away for long, not least because he or she needs to discover and use them. The easiest way to trim

A bath thermometer takes the guesswork out of bathing your baby, but you should still double-check the temperature of the water with your elbow.

Topping and tailing

Clean your baby in a warm room, so that exposed skin doesn't get cold. You can use a changing table, a bed or sofa, or the floor, but cover the surface with a thick towel folded over a few times to keep the baby warm and comfortable. Either undress the baby completely and cover with a towel to keep warm, or remove clothing as you go along. Never leave your baby unattended on a raised surface, even if you think he or she can't yet roll over. Get everything ready before you start: you'll need a bowl of warm boiled water, cotton wool (cotton balls), a facecloth, a small, thin towel and a clean nappy (plus nappy rash cream, if necessary).

1 Cover the baby's lower half with a towel. Dip a small wad of cotton wool in the water, and wipe the baby's eye from the inner to the outer corner. Use a new piece of damp cotton wool to clean the other eye.

2 Use more wet cotton wool or a clean, damp facecloth to wipe the baby's face, including the nose and ears. Clean the folds of the neck (dried milk can collect here) and pat the baby dry with a clean towel.

3 Move the towel to cover the baby's top half. Now clean the nappy area, make sure you wipe all the folds in the legs and groin. Do not pull back a boy's foreskin or a girl's labia – these areas are self-cleaning. Pat dry.

Bathing

You can bath your baby in an ordinary bath, but using a baby bath is more convenient and uses less water. You can use a baby bath inside an ordinary bath, but it will be less strain on your back if you place it on the floor, or, better yet, on a stand. Make sure that the room is very warm before you undress the baby, and always check the temperature of the bathwater before immersing the baby in it. It's easier to get the right temperature if you fill the bath with warm water and then gradually add cold. Keep baths very short – a few minutes is all that is necessary – and hold the baby firmly to help him or her feel secure. It will be reassuring if you talk in a low, calm tone.

1 Undress your baby and wrap in a towel, leaving the head exposed. Hold the baby over the bath, supporting the back, neck and head with one arm and hand. Use the other hand to wash the baby's hair with water (there's no need for shampoo). Gently pat dry.

2 Remove the towel and lower your baby into the bath, holding under the arm with your hand and supporting the neck and head with your wrist. Support the bottom with your other hand. Continue to support the baby's back and neck while you use the other hand to rinse.

3 Lift the baby out and lay him or her on a towel, quickly wrapping it around him or her, covering the head as well as the body (a hooded towel works best). Dry well, all over, including the creases, and then put on a clean nappy and sleepsuit.

---

nails is to use baby clippers. Do it after a bath when the nails are softer, or when the baby is asleep. Hold the finger between your thumb and forefinger, and press the pad out of the way while you clip. You can also use a nail file, which doesn't leave sharp edges, or you can nibble your baby's nails short. Fingernails grow quickly, so check them every couple of days. Toenails should be trimmed in the same way, but they grow more slowly so won't need doing so often.

Trim your baby's nails when he or she is asleep, or is at least calm and still. Make sure there is enough light to see by – it is very easy to nick the skin by accident. Use baby nail clippers rather than scissors.

BATH SUPPORT

A framed towelling bath support makes bathing your baby much easier, since it leaves both your hands free and supports the baby's head. When your baby is a few weeks old, it will help to make bath time more enjoyable for you both. The towelling can become chilly when it is wet, so keep scooping water over it.

Caring for your baby's skin

Baby skin is very delicate and can easily become dry. The best way to protect it is to treat it as naturally as possible, and minimize any contact with chemicals. For example, use a soap-based washing powder rather than a detergent (biological ones are definitely to be avoided). Do not use fabric softeners, which can irritate a baby's skin. Always wash new clothing before putting it on your baby, since the fabric may contain chemicals left over from the manufacturing process. Where possible, choose clothes made from organic fabrics, such as cotton. Unbleached, undyed fabrics are the best choice for bedding and clothing that will be next to your baby's skin.

SKINCARE AT BATHTIME
It takes a few weeks for the oils in the skin of a newborn baby to form a natural protective barrier, so it is a good idea to avoid bathing your baby during this time: top and tail instead. Restrict baths to no more than two or three a week and don't use any baby bath products, especially those that contain petrochemicals, alcohol or perfume. Your baby is unlikely to get so dirty that he or she needs washing with soap, and you won't need baby shampoo for months – water will do the job all on its own.

It's fine to add the very gentle essential oils of Roman chamomile and lavender to a baby's bath so long as he or she is three months or more. Use one or two drops, diluted in oil or full fat milk before added to the water.

A baby's skin has a gorgeous natural scent. Perfumed bubble baths and other products aren't necessary.

Bathing in oatmeal
An oatmeal bath is an excellent way to soften and moisturize babies' delicate skin. It can also be used to help relieve the itching associated with eczema, chickenpox or insect bites.

1 Grind two cups of oatmeal in a clean coffee grinder, blender or food processor until it is very fine. Combine the ground oatmeal with four cups of cold water, stirring well.

2 Add the oatmeal solution to a tepid bath – the water should look slightly milky and feel slimy to the touch (if the oatmeal drops to the bottom of the bathtub, it hasn't been ground finely enough).

3 Take care not to get any water in the baby's eyes during the bath since the oatmeal can irritate. You also need to be very careful when holding or lifting your baby because this bath makes skin extremely slippery.

BABY MASSAGE OIL

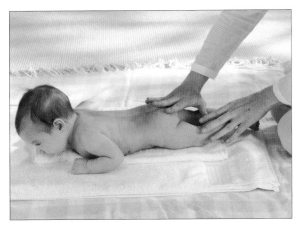

Oiling or moisturizing your baby's skin after every bath will help to keep it soft and hydrated. Using oil will also allow you to massage your baby without pulling the skin. But make sure that all the creases are completely dry before applying oil or you'll be creating the ideal conditions for fungal infection. You can use lavender and Roman chamomile essential oils on babies of three months or older. If your baby was born prematurely, wait until at least three months after your due date.

100ml (3½fl oz) sunflower oil
5 drops lavender essential oil
5 drops Roman chamomile essential oil

Pour the sunflower oil into a dark glass bottle then add the essential oils. Replace the cap and shake well to mix. When using for massage, pour a small amount on your hands and rub your palms together, then smooth over your baby's skin. Add more oil whenever you notice that the skin is starting to pull.

Plain water can be drying, so it is worth adding a little oil to the water to help keep your baby's skin soft and supple. Many parents like to use almond or jojoba oil in their babies' baths. But a few babies can react to nut-based oils such as these, so it may be safer to stick with vegetable oils like sunflower or olive at first. Alternatively, you can use oatmeal in the bath, which is a natural emollient.

CRADLE CAP

Lots of babies develop thick yellowish scales on their scalp. This happens when the sebaceous glands in the skin produce too much sebum, the oily substance that helps to keep skin lubricated. Cradle cap doesn't do any

Cradle cap can last for many months if you don't treat it. Smoothing olive oil into the scalp is a simple remedy.

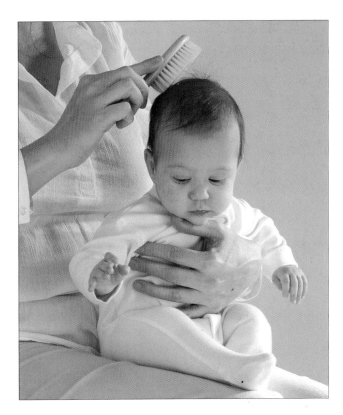

Use a baby brush, with very soft bristles, to help clear off the loose scales of cradle cap.

harm, but it can look unsightly and may persist for months if you don't treat it. To do so, gently rub some olive oil into the area and leave overnight, then wash off in the morning. To help cradle cap on its way, you can brush the scalp with a baby hairbrush to remove loose scales. Never pick off scales with your fingers or you may cause infection. If the cradle cap is very stubborn, try rubbing in calendula cream every night for a few days.

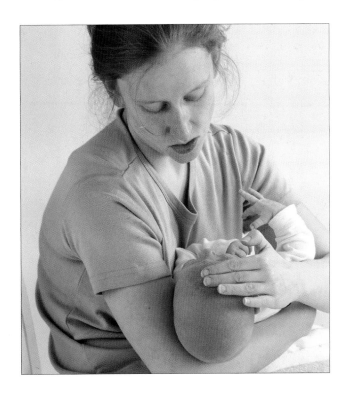

Clothes for your baby

Babies are not good at regulating their body temperature, so they must always be dressed appropriately for the weather. On a hot day, a nappy and perhaps a vest may be all your baby needs. On cold days, a vest, an all-in-one towelling sleepsuit and a light cardigan should be sufficient. Be ready to change your baby's clothing if the temperature changes or you go out.

You can tell if a baby is warm enough by feeling the back of the neck. If it is cold, you need to put on more clothing. But don't worry if the baby's hands and feet feel cooler than the rest of the body; this is quite normal. To check if a baby is getting too hot, feel the tummy or chest. Remove a layer of clothing if the skin is very warm.

Choose clothes made from fabric that is soft, stretchable and machine-washable – cotton is ideal. And make sure that everything is easy to put on and take off. You'll find all-in-ones with roomy necklines and snap fasteners a lot less restricting than denim jackets or party frocks. Shoes may look cute on a baby, but they can cramp the feet and restrict growth if they are too tight. It is much better to let your baby go barefoot so that he or she can wriggle his or her toes freely, or to put him or her in soft socks or tights to keep the feet warm. Make sure there is plenty of "wriggle room" in the socks, and cut the feet off sleepsuits once they get snug in the feet.

BABY BASICS

Some of the most useful basic items of clothes for a young baby that will help you to have what you need whatever the weather are as follows.

If it is hot, your baby may not need to wear any clothes at all. Some young babies feel insecure if they are naked and prefer to wear a vest, but most soon love the feeling of being bare.

Six short-sleeved bodysuits or vests. These may be all your baby needs to wear on summer days, and they make useful undergarments in winter. Long-sleeved bodysuits are good for winter but are harder to get on.
Six to eight long-sleeved sleepsuits with feet. Great as pyjamas or daywear for young babies, but make sure they are roomy enough in the feet. You'll need fewer in

Lots of parents tend to overdress their babies. On a warm day, or in a centrally heated house, a bodysuit or vest on top of the nappy may be all he or she needs to stay comfortable.

Baby clothes have to be simple and practical. Frills, fiddly buttons and fussy necklines all make dressing your baby hard work, and synthetic fabrics may irritate the skin and cause overheating.

Putting clothes on your baby

Many babies hate having their clothes changed, so do it only when their clothing is soiled or wet – there's no need to put a baby into a different sleepsuit for the night, say, if the one he or she has on is perfectly clean. Make sure the room is warm, especially in the early months, and place the baby on a comfortable surface. Work as gently and as quickly as possible, without getting flustered (it gets easier with practice). If the baby seems worried or distressed when naked, lay a small towel over him or her to give a greater feeling of security.

It will help if you maintain eye contact with your baby and sing or chat as you dress him or her. With an older baby, you can turn dressing into a game – play peek-a-boo as you pull a sleepsuit over your baby's face.

1 When putting on a vest or bodysuit, use your hands to stretch the neck as wide as possible. This will help you to ease it over the baby's head without scraping the nose or ears. Do this as quickly as possible since babies don't like having their faces covered.

2 If the garment has long sleeves, gather the sleeve fabric as close to the armhole as possible. Put your fingers through, gently hold your baby's hand and pull the sleeve over the arm rather than tugging a tiny arm through the sleeve. Repeat with the other arm.

3 To put on an all-in-one sleepsuit, open up all the fastenings and lay the suit on a flat changing surface. Place the baby on top. Gently ease the feet of the suit over your baby's feet. Pull the sleeves over the arms as before. Do up the fastenings from the feet upwards.

summer, when it may be too hot for the baby to wear them during the day.

Two to three cardigans. These are much easier to put on than garments that go over the head, but choose the kind that fasten with snaps rather than fiddly buttons.

Baby blanket. Good for wrapping the baby up when you need to go outside, or for use as a cover during naps.

Baby sleeping bag. A great alternative to blankets, which can be kicked off, a sleeping bag is a good way to make sure your baby stays warm. Combine a sleeping bag with a long-sleeved bodysuit, and add a cardigan if it is very cold. You can get bags with lighter tog ratings suitable for summer.

Three to six bibs. Useful if your baby spits up milk after feeds, or is dribbling a lot because of teething.

One or two hats. For summer, choose cotton hats with a wide, floppy brim (especially important if you are using a sling and need to protect the top of the baby's head). For winter, buy hats that are made of fleece or similar, with flaps that go over the ears.

Two to six pairs of socks. Get them all in the same colour, as you are bound to lose quite a few. You won't need many in summer.

Snowsuit with built-in mittens. This is great for keeping a baby cosy when you go out in winter. But you won't need one if you have a warm inner sleeve for the buggy or if you are carrying your baby in a sling; choose a cape or warm coat instead.

Babies should normally have their heads uncovered when they are indoors, but very small, or premature, babies may need to wear a hat in the first few days. Check with your midwife if you are unsure what is best.

Out and about

Going out with a young baby can feel quite stressful at first, so it is a good idea to keep trips short and relatively simple until you get used to the outside world again. Carrying your baby in a sling will help you both feel secure but can be hard on your back. Sooner or later you will need a buggy. Choose one that lies flat or use a pram for the first few months to avoid putting pressure on the baby's developing spine. A buggy with a seat that faces you will allow you to keep an eye on a young baby, and means he or she has your reassuring presence in view.

When you go out, your baby will need to wear extra layers and a hat (body heat can rapidly escape through the top of the head). To avoid overheating, you should take off any outer clothing and remove blankets and rain covers when you come back indoors or if you go into a warm shop or café, even if it means waking your baby up. Rain

It is important to keep a young baby out of direct sunlight at all times. A wide-brimmed hat will help to shade his or her face.

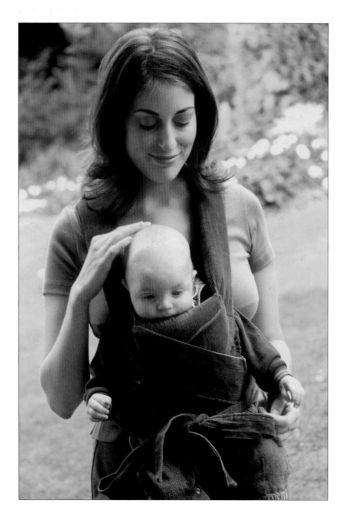

Slings seem fiddly, with lots of straps and buckles to work out, but they are very comfortable and your baby will love being close to you.

CHECKLIST: PACKING YOUR DAY BAG

It is worth investing in a proper changing bag, which is designed to carry everything you need for a day out. Write out your own list and keep it in the bag so that you can check you have everything whenever you go out.

- Nappies (diapers) and cotton wool (cotton balls)
- Flask of boiled water, or alcohol-free wipes
- Nappy sacks
- Nappy rash cream
- Complete change of clothes
- Muslins to protect your clothing and clean up baby
- Bottles of formula or expressed breastmilk, if using
- Bottle of cooled, boiled water, if using
- Snacks for breastfeeding mother
- Comforter or dummy (pacifier), if using
- One or two toys

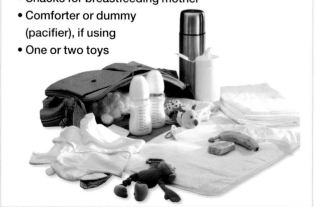

Take outdoor clothing off your baby when you enter a warm building. If the baby is asleep it is tempting not to do this, but he or she could become overheated.

covers and sunshades trap warm air around your baby, so be sure to open ventilation flaps whenever possible, and put covers and shades down when you go indoors. Using a UV-filter sunshade will keep your baby cooler than the buggy hood, and will give more protection from sunlight.

SUN PROTECTION

Babies under six months old should not be exposed to direct sunlight because their skin is too thin to protect them from harmful UV rays. Put a sunhat with a wide brim on a baby who is being carried in a sling, and cover arms and legs completely with a cool fabric such as cotton. If your baby is in a buggy, get a parasol and adjust it frequently so that your baby is kept in the shade. This is much easier if the baby is facing you; if your buggy faces away from you (as most do), a UV-filter sunshade will be more effective.

CHOOSING A CAR SEAT

It is essential that you use the right type of car seat for your baby, even if you need it only for short trips. A car seat is one baby item that you should definitely buy new, unless it comes from somebody that you know and trust, and you are certain that it has not been involved in an accident. You cannot always tell from the appearance of a car seat whether or not it has been damaged, so it is risky to use one from an unknown source.

For the first nine months or so, babies need a backward-facing car seat. This helps to protect their undeveloped neck muscles from a whiplash-type injury, which would be much more serious than in an adult. Choose one that has high sides to protect from side-impact blows. Once your baby weighs 9kg/20lb or more and can sit unsupported for at least 15 minutes, he or she can go in a forward-facing seat.

A travel cot provides your baby with a safe place to sleep wherever you are.

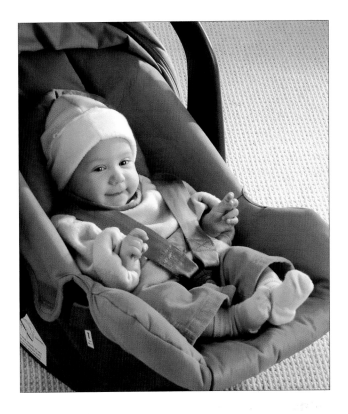

LEAVING HOME

Going away with your baby can be a daunting prospect, especially when you start to think about how much you need to take with you. But it's actually easier when a baby is very small, especially if you are breastfeeding. Here is a list of some of the things you may need.

SLEEPING
- Travel cot or Moses basket (unless your baby sleeps with you)
- Fitted sheet and flat sheet
- Blankets or baby sleeping bag
- Any sleep aids you may have been using (such as CDs or comforters)

CLOTHING
- Three complete changes for each day (fewer if you have washing facilities), and outdoor clothing
- Bibs, if using
- One or two baby towels

FEEDING
- Formula, bottles and teats, if using
- Sterilizer, if using (if you have access to a kitchen, you can boil bottles and teats in a large saucepan instead)

OTHER ITEMS
- Baby bouncer or play mat, if using
- Selection of toys (including any that your baby has grown attached to)
- Change of clothing for you
- Sling or buggy, if using, for going out and about

Why breastfeed?

Breastfeeding involves more than simply giving your baby milk. Snuggled at your breast, your baby enjoys your warmth, your scent and the familiar sound of your heartbeat. He or she can gaze upon your face, which is just the right distance away to focus on. Your baby is blissfully content. Before the birth, lots of women worry about whether they will be able to breastfeed their child. But almost everyone can, provided that they have a supportive environment in which to do it. And although you may experience some difficulties along the way, nursing can be as satisfying and loving an experience for you as it is for your baby.

SUCCESSFUL BREASTFEEDING

One of the keys to successful breastfeeding is simply trusting that you can do it. In societies where breastfeeding is the only safe way to nourish infants, new mothers assume that they can breastfeed – and they do. After all, our bodies are designed to nurture our babies both before and after birth.

Good support boosts your confidence and encourages you to continue through any initial problems. Studies have found that having a partner who is positive about breastfeeding can have a major effect. The support of friends and relatives, particularly women who have successfully breastfed themselves, can also make a big difference. It is well worth seeking out a breastfeeding counsellor or an organization such as La Leche League, who may run a drop-in support group in your area.

WHAT IS BREASTMILK?

Breastmilk is the perfect food for babies. It provides the nutrients they need in exactly the right quantities and it is packed with antibodies to help them fight off infection and illness. It is also completely sterile. Unlike formula milk, breastmilk is a living substance that adapts to your baby's needs. It varies from day to day, and from feed to feed. For example, it may contain specific antibodies to help your baby fight off any germs you encountered that day and it will have a higher water content on hot days. It is usually denser in the morning, after you have rested.

The first milk you produce is colostrum, rich in antibodies and nutrients, and with laxative properties that encourage your baby to pass the sticky first stools (meconium). True breastmilk comes in a few days after the birth. Each feed begins with thin foremilk to quench

Fathers have a role in breastfeeding too: a supportive partner can be a key factor in successful breastfeeding, as can friends and relatives.

Nursing is an expression of love that only a mother can give. A baby who is upset or ill instinctively turns to you for the comfort of nursing.

Breastfeeding not only gives a baby a feeling of security and comfort, it also has a soothing effect on the mother, and gives her a reason to relax and rest.

Even if you don't intend to breastfeed for long, nursing your baby for the first few days will give him or her some level of protection from infections.

the baby's thirst. As the baby continues sucking, denser hindmilk is produced. This is high in fat and proteins and gives your baby the energy he or she needs to grow.

THE ADVANTAGES OF BREASTFEEDING

It's more convenient. It is much easier to breastfeed than to prepare and warm a bottle, especially in the middle of the night.

It's better for your baby. Breastfed babies suffer from fewer tummy bugs than bottle-fed ones (one study found that American bottle-fed babies got diarrhoea more than 12 times more often). They also get half as many colds and are less likely to get respiratory diseases and ear and urine infections.

It sets the foundations for good health in adult life. Breastfeeding exclusively for six months helps protect your baby from allergies. Breastfed babies are less likely to be obese in later life, or to develop eczema, diabetes and high blood pressure. There is also evidence to suggest breastfeeding helps with brain development.

It encourages the development of the jaw and teeth. Breastfed babies may have fewer dental problems.

It exposes your baby to a wide range of tastes. The flavour of breastmilk varies depending on what you eat. This may help with weaning.

It is enjoyable. Babies nurse for comfort as well as food, and breastfeeding is the quickest way to calm a baby who is distressed.

It helps you to get back in shape. Breastfeeding stimulates the production of oxytocin, which helps your womb return to its normal size. And the fat stores you laid down in pregnancy are used in producing your milk.

It helps you to relax. You have to sit down to nurse

your baby, which means you rest. Also, nursing mothers have higher levels of the hormone prolactin. This helps you to feel calm, so you can sleep quickly after a feed.

It has benefits for your health. Breastfeeding may reduce the chances of developing breast or ovarian cancer, and lower the risk of osteoporosis.

It delays the return of your periods. Breastfeeding has a contraceptive effect and you are unlikely to become pregnant if you are feeding on demand and do not go longer than four hours between any feeds. But if you need to be certain of avoiding pregnancy, you should use another method of contraception.

VITAMIN D

There is some debate about whether breastfed babies get enough vitamin D, which is important for bone health. It is present in breastmilk in low amounts and is manufactured in the skin when exposed to sunlight. Since we are now advised to protect babies from the sun, they are more reliant on breastmilk for their supply. The American Academy of Pediatrics recommends that all breastfed babies are given vitamin D drops as a precaution, while the UK Department of Health advises vitamin D (as well as C and A) for babies of six months and over who still have breastmilk as their main drink.

Whether or not your baby needs drops may depend on where you live and, to an extent, on the colour of your skin (dark-skinned babies are at greater risk of vitamin D deficiency). It is worth talking to a health professional about what is best for your baby.

Feeding on demand

Your breasts will almost certainly produce as much milk as your baby needs, provided that you feed as often and for as long as the baby wants to. In the first weeks, this may mean you are feeding 10–12 times a day so that it feels like nursing is an almost permanent activity. You may find it hard to believe that your baby can be hungry so quickly after the last feed. But a baby's tiny stomach – about the size of a walnut – can take in only a small amount of milk at a time. Breastmilk is so easily digested that it doesn't remain there for long.

If babies get less than they need at a feed, whether it's because they go to sleep, or feed very slowly, they will want to nurse again sooner. By allowing your baby to nurse as soon as he or she is hungry, your breasts get the message that more milk is needed and will adjust their supply accordingly. It may take anything from a few days to a few weeks, but eventually your baby will start to go longer between feeds.

Every so often, you'll notice that your baby suddenly wants to feed more frequently again. These increases in demand often happen at around two weeks, six weeks

Lots of babies come off the breast when they are satisfied, but some like to go to sleep with their mother's nipple in their mouth. You may find that your baby wakes and cries when you remove it. If so, try letting the baby suckle once more and then taking him or her off again. You may have to do this several times before the baby will relinquish your nipple.

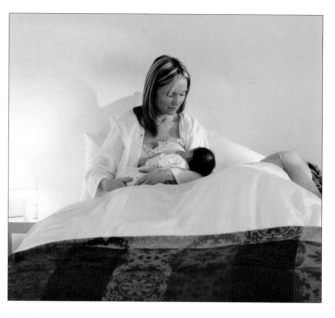

Feeding your baby on demand can be tough at first – most women find that they are nursing four or five times a night. But you get used to going back to sleep quickly, and eventually your baby will wake less often.

and 12 weeks, and indicate growth spurts. Again, if you let the baby nurse on demand, your milk supply will increase to meet his or her needs. Mothers often wonder how long a feed should last. The answer, annoyingly, is that it varies depending on how your baby feeds. Some babies keep sucking vigorously until they are satisfied, and they may get enough milk in 10–15 minutes. Others tend to feed in short bursts, resting in between. It may take an hour or more for them to feel sated. With slow feeders, it can sometimes feel as if one feed rolls into the next. There isn't a lot you can do about this: just accept that for now you will be spending most of the time nursing. Babies gradually become more efficient at feeding, so your feeds will get shorter.

EARLY BOTTLES

Don't give your baby any bottles of formula early on: if your baby is getting nourishment elsewhere, he or she will feed less often at the breast – and your milk supply won't increase in the way it needs to. Also, it requires less work for a baby to get milk from the teat of a bottle than the nipple, so if you give a bottle, the baby may refuse breastfeeds altogether. If you want to combine breast and bottle-feeding it is still best to breastfeed exclusively for six weeks to establish the milk supply. It is also best to avoid using a dummy (pacifier) during this time.

ONE SIDE OR TWO?

Mothers are sometimes advised to feed from each breast for a specific time. But if you do this, your baby may get only the thin foremilk, so you need to let the baby suckle at one breast for as long as he or she wants. If this empties the breast (which will then feel soft rather than full) but the baby still seems to be hungry, offer the other one. For the next feed, offer the second breast first, so the feeds start on alternate sides. To help you remember which side to start on, try attaching a safety pin or ribbon to your bra strap and moving it to the opposite side at each feed. Some women find that they can tell which breast to start on, because it is heavier.

IS IT WORKING?

The number of wet nappies produced can be the best indicator of whether your baby is getting enough milk: if there are fewer than six a day, you may need to check your latching-on technique or look at ways of boosting your milk supply. Make sure you are resting enough and drinking enough fluids. A baby mustn't be dehydrated, so talk to a health professional if you are worried.

If your baby is gaining weight slowly or in a different way to the development charts babies are measured against, don't assume you are not feeding successfully. It is normal for babies to lose up to 10 per cent of their birth weight in the first week, and to grow less in some weeks than in others. So long as they gain weight steadily over a number of weeks, they are probably feeding enough.

Like any new skill, breastfeeding takes practice and you may want to give yourself privacy at first. But once you and your baby get the hang of it, you can nurse discreetly without other people taking much notice.

Breastmilk continues to have health benefits even after a baby is on solid food. Many women continue breastfeeding for two years or more.

HOW LONG TO BREASTFEED

Ideally, women would breastfeed their babies exclusively for six months and then continue to nurse for at least the first year, even after solids have been introduced.

Lots of women give up breastfeeding if they suffer from sore nipples or other problems early on. This is a shame, because breastfeeding usually gets much easier, quicker and more satisfying for the mother once the baby is a little older. You may find that you are able to go on longer than you expected, particularly if you get support and seek out other women who are breastfeeding for encouragement.

A hungry baby may cry, nuzzle against your breast or make rooting or sucking movements. Try to feed a hungry baby as soon as possible. Any period of breastfeeding will benefit your baby, so it is definitely worth starting, even if you don't think you will want to continue for very long.

Breastfeeding basics

Your baby will instinctively search for your nipple with an open mouth when placed on the breast (this is the rooting reflex that all babies are born with). But you need to give your baby some help to make sure he or she takes your breast in a way that enables him or her to get as much milk as is needed as efficiently as possible. It is also important that the feeding process doesn't make your nipples sore. This can be tricky at first, but with practice you and your baby will achieve the correct latch each time with ease. When a baby is latched on correctly, his or her gums press on the areola (the dark bit around the nipple) and stimulate the milk ducts inside the breast. As the baby sucks, the gums act in the same way as a pump, drawing milk into the nipple. The sucking also sets off the mother's "let-down reflex" in the breast, which pushes milk from the production glands and into the milk glands.

WHAT NOT TO DO
- Don't put your hand behind the baby's head and pull it towards you. The baby will arch away.
- Don't position your nipple opposite the baby's mouth. Make sure that it is in line with the nose, or the baby won't be able to draw it deeply enough into the mouth.
- Don't press on your breast to make an airspace for the baby's nose – you could cause a blockage in a milk duct or move the nipple out of position. If the nose is squashed, try moving the baby's bottom closer to your body to create space.
- Don't continue if you feel pain that lasts more than a few seconds. Take the baby off and start again.

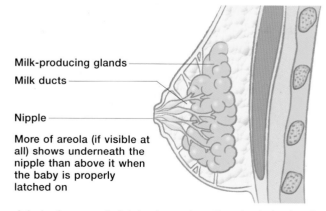

Milk-producing glands

Milk ducts

Nipple

More of areola (if visible at all) shows underneath the nipple than above it when the baby is properly latched on

A baby is properly latched on when the nipple is deeply inside the mouth. The tongue should be beneath the nipple, while the gums clamp down behind it.

LATCHING ON
As the baby sucks you should be able to see the jaw and ears moving and hear swallowing. If you can hear smacking sounds or the baby's cheeks are drawing in, he or she is not latched on properly.

1 Hold the baby close to you, tummy against yours and nose opposite your nipple. Make sure the baby is completely on his or her side, with head, shoulders and back forming a straight line. Support your breast with your fingers, keeping them clear of the areola. Your baby may open his or her mouth and reach towards the nipple. If not, brush the baby's lower lip with your nipple.

2 As the baby's mouth opens very wide, gently draw the shoulders towards you so that the baby can take the nipple and as much as possible of the areola into the mouth. The gums should close well clear of the nipple. If you feel discomfort for more than a few seconds, wet your little finger and slip it into the side of the baby's mouth to release the suction. Take the baby off the breast, then try again.

YOUR POSITION

You can breastfeed sitting down, leaning back, lying on your side or even standing up. All that matters is that the baby is in the right position for latching on and that you are comfortable and relaxed. You shouldn't have to lean or hunch over in order to get the breast in the baby's mouth – use pillows to support your back and the arm you are using to hold the baby, and put your feet up.

Cradle hold: The baby's head rests on your forearm, just below the crook of your arm, with his or her body supported along your forearm and bottom in your hand. Make sure you are tummy-to-tummy and place the baby's lower arm around your waist. This position is good for women comfortable with breastfeeding.

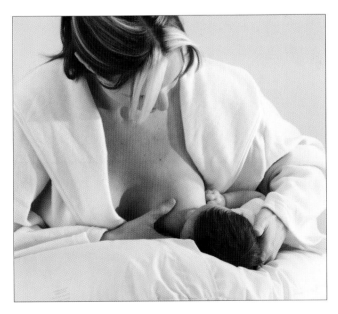

Clutch hold: Tuck the baby under your arm, facing you. The baby's head and shoulders are held in your hand, the back is supported by your forearm and the legs rest on a pillow behind you. This position allows you to guide the baby's head to your breast easily, so it is a good one to start with. It can be used if you've had a Caesarean, and also makes it possible to nurse twins simultaneously.

Lying-down position: You and the baby lie on your sides facing each other (put pillows under your head, behind your back and between your knees for extra support). Raise your lower arm above your head or use it to cradle the baby's shoulders and head. This position works well for night feeds but some women find it a bit tricky at first.

BURPING

Babies take in air when they feed and often need to burp afterwards. If your baby has fallen asleep feeding, you don't need to wake him or her to burp, but there may be one later. Some babies don't burp straight away so keep patting or change position, but if your baby doesn't burp after a while, then he or she probably doesn't need to.

The simplest burping position involves holding the baby against your shoulder and gently rubbing or patting the back for a few minutes.

Alternatively, sit the baby on your knee, supporting the chin. Lean his or her chest on one hand and rub his or her back with the other.

Breast care and expressing

Even if you have breastfed a baby before, it can take your breasts some time to adapt to all the extra stimulation that they are getting. There is a lot you can do to prevent discomfort in the early weeks. Make sure you wear a proper nursing bra that fits properly. Most women find their breasts are a cup size bigger when their milk comes in, and a bra that is too small may cause your milk ducts to become blocked. You need three or four bras. Air your breasts often. If they are covered up whenever you are not feeding, warmth and moisture can build up, creating the ideal conditions for fungal infection. So expose your breasts to the air after every feed.

Don't wash your nipples with anything other than water – soap can be very drying and may encourage cracking. After each feed, rub a little breastmilk over the nipple and areola to keep them lubricated. Let them dry naturally. Eat

Wear loose, comfortable clothes that can be easily adjusted for feeding, especially in the first few weeks.

healthily and frequently. Breastfeeding women need an extra 500 calories a day, more if nursing twins. It is very important not to diet, since this will affect your milk supply and reduce your energy. Drink lots of water. Most women get very thirsty when they are nursing. Have a large bottle of water next to you when you feed, and drink regularly at other times too.

Breast pads protect your bra and clothing from leaking. You can get washable, reusable, unbleached ones, which are more environmentally friendly than the disposable sort. Plastic breast shells to collect the milk are helpful when expressing, or if your breast leaks a great deal when your baby is on the other nipple.

WHAT TO EAT

Both you and the baby will benefit if you have a healthy diet. Your daily requirements for vitamins and minerals go up when you are breastfeeding, but you can easily meet them by eating at least five portions of fruits and vegetables a day, plus whole grains, dairy foods or other calcium-rich foods, oily and white fish, lean meat, pulses and nuts. A balanced diet includes some fat, which you can get from healthy sources such as avocado, olive and vegetable oil, and oily fish.

EXPRESSING MILK

Before you had your baby, you may have assumed that you would express often so that your partner could feed while you rested. In reality you may find that you have neither the time nor the inclination to express. But if your

Your breasts may feel hard, hot and swollen when your milk first comes in. To relieve this, place a Savoy cabbage leaf, scored at the stem, inside each bra cup

---

CAUTION
Do not take any prescription or over-the-counter drugs without checking that they are safe for nursing mothers. Check with your pharmacist or doctor.

baby is in special care, if you develop very sore or cracked nipples or if you have to go back to work, then expressing can be indispensable. There are three methods: by hand, by hand pump or by electric pump. Electric pumps tend to give the fastest results, but some women prefer a hand pump. Hand expressing is much slower, but it requires no equipment and can work very well for women who have a fast milk flow. If you know that you will need your baby to take a bottle, give expressed milk once a week from about six weeks.

STORING YOUR MILK
Expressed breastmilk can be stored in a completely clean, sterilized feeding bottle. Keep the bottle in the middle of the refrigerator (not in the door) for up to 24 hours. If you want to keep it longer, it is best to freeze it. When you are planning to use frozen milk, take it out of

Electric breastpumps tend to be easier to use than hand ones. But expressing is a knack so don't worry if you get only a few drops at first.

FOOD AND DRINKS TO LIMIT OR AVOID
- Do not eat peanuts or peanut products if you, the father or close relatives of either of you suffer from hay fever, eczema, asthma or other allergies.
- Limit shark, fresh swordfish, marlin and fresh tuna to no more than one portion a week, and canned tuna to two cans a week. These fish contain traces of mercury.
- Cut out any foods that seem to upset your baby. Some babies react if their mothers eat spicy foods, citrus fruit or cows' milk. But don't feel you need to avoid such foods as a precautionary measure since very few babies are affected in this way.
- Avoid or at least restrict your intake of caffeine-rich drinks (coffee, tea, cola), since these can unsettle the baby.
- Do not drink much alcohol. An occasional glass of wine or beer should do no harm, but limit yourself to no more than one glass in a day and avoid drinking just before you feed your baby. The level of alcohol in your milk will drop over time, so if possible wait two hours before feeding again.

the freezer and place in the fridge to defrost for 12 hours. If you need it in a hurry, place the bottle in a bowl of hot water. Do not refreeze defrosted breastmilk.

One of the advantages of introducing a bottle feed is that fathers can take part in the profound bonding experience of feeding their baby.

Expressing by hand
Place warm flannels on your breasts or take a warm shower to encourage your milk to flow. Take a few moments to relax. Think about and look at your baby, or look at a photograph, to stimulate the let-down reflex.

1 Supporting your breast with one hand, use the other to stroke from the top of the breast to the nipple. Do this for 30 seconds or so, and be very gentle.

2 Cup the breast with your thumb and forefinger, placing them at the outer edge of the areola. Use a rhythmic squeeze and release motion, pushing your thumb and fingers slightly backwards (towards the chest wall) at the same time, until drops of milk appear.

3 Lean forward slightly so that you can collect the milk in a sterilized container as you continue to squeeze and release. Move your hand around the edge of the areola, so that you empty the breast. When the flow of milk slows, switch to the other breast. Repeat on both sides.

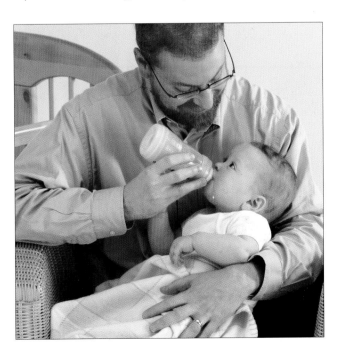

Common problems for nursing mothers

Breastfeeding problems often occur when a new mother is trying to do too much. So the best response is to take yourself off to bed for a couple of days with your baby. Ask someone else to take care of food and any chores so that you can concentrate on nursing. Frequent feeding and lots of rest can do a lot to help.

SORE NIPPLES

The problem new mothers complain about most – and with good reason – is sore nipples. Usually, soreness is due to incorrect positioning at the breast, so the best way to avoid it is to ensure that your baby is latched on properly every time. Rest assured that your nipples won't be sore all the time that you breastfeed – they will adjust and you will find latching on easier. In the meantime, you can help yourself in the following ways.

- Gently rub breastmilk over the nipple area after each feed and let it dry naturally. Airing the breasts regularly will also encourage healing – go topless when at home.
- Use lanolin cream to soften the nipples and heal any cracking. Calendula cream can also be used, but you need to wash off any residue before nursing your baby.
- Take the homeopathic remedy Castor equi.
- Do not restrict feeds, as this can cause the baby to grip the breast and suck harder.
- If all else fails, use nipple shields. These plastic caps cover the nipple while feeding. Some experts advise against using them because they can make it harder for your baby to suck, but they can be a good temporary

If you get a blocked duct, sore nipples or other breastfeeding problem, it may be a sign that you are doing too much. Spending one or two days in bed or on the sofa with your baby may be all you need to do.

measure if you are in pain, especially if the nipple is cracked. If milk collects behind the shield after your baby has been on the breast for a few minutes, then he or she is probably getting enough.

THRUSH

Occasionally, painful nipples may be due to the fungal infection thrush. If you have thrush, your nipples are likely to be red and itchy, and there may be white patches on them. In addition, you may be able to see white patches in the baby's mouth. You will both need to be treated, otherwise you will keep reinfecting each other.

The pain of thrush can make it hard to breastfeed, so it is important to treat it promptly. See your doctor for some antifungal gel: you spread it on your nipples and in the baby's mouth.

Occasionally, women get thrush in the milk ducts (which causes breast pain). This needs an oral antifungal treatment. It is also a good idea to take acidophilus supplements or eat bio-active yogurt to restore the "good" bacteria in your system: this keeps the thrush fungus naturally under control. You can also get a probiotic suitable for young babies from good health food stores. Some women find it helps to cut out sugar and yeast for a while.

Arm swinging can help with blocked ducts or engorgement because it gets your milk flowing.

Thrush thrives in warm damp areas, so rinse your breasts after feeding (use plain water or a solution of one tablespoon vinegar in one cup of water) and expose to the air until dry. Be vigilant about hygiene: wash your hands with soap after using the toilet, before and after changing a nappy, and after feeding while treatment is ongoing. Use paper towels to dry your hands and discard; wash bath towels after each use in hot water (if possible, add a little white vinegar to the final rinse) Wash any toys or dummies in hot soapy water, then boil for 15 minutes.

BLOCKED DUCTS

If a milk duct becomes blocked, you'll notice a small hard lump in the breast. This may not hurt, but you need to clear it since an infection could develop, leading to mastitis. A blocked duct can be caused by a tight bra or by pressing your breast with a finger to make room for the baby's nose. It is often the result of the baby being latched on wrongly, so that some of the milk ducts are not being emptied. To treat a blocked duct:

- Change your bra or stop pressing on the breast.
- Apply warm flannels to the area before and between feeds. Some women find cold compresses (a packet of frozen peas wrapped in a small towel makes a good one) more helpful.
- Feed often (express if your baby is unwilling).
- Try an alternative feeding position so that your baby drains the breast from a different direction.
- While feeding, very gently stroke your fingers over the area and towards the nipple.
- Try arm circles before a feed, to help the milk flow.

MASTITIS

If a blockage is not cleared, then part of the breast can become inflamed. You will see a hot, red patch on the breast, which will feel hard. This is the early stage of mastitis. If it is left untreated, you will also get a high temperature and feel very ill (as if you have flu). If you

Mastitis starts with a hot, red patch on the breast. If you catch it early on, you may be able to avoid antibiotics.

react quickly enough, you may be able to treat mastitis by resting for a day or two (preferably in bed with your baby) and by following the advice for clearing a blocked duct. It is very important to keep feeding, and it is helpful to express any milk left in the breast after a feed to ensure that the breast is completely drained. A homeopath may recommend Belladonna or Hepar sulph, or you may want to take painkillers such as paracetamol (acetaminophen). See your doctor if you do not start to feel better after a day or so, or if you feel worse despite self-help measures.

If the mastitis is due to an infection in the breast, then it is best to take antibiotics to clear it. If it is left untreated, you may get a breast abscess. Many doctors recommend antibiotics at the first sign of mastitis. Most antibiotics are safe to take when you are breastfeeding, but they may cause your baby to become irritable or to produce stools that are looser than normal. To avoid another bout, be vigilant about positioning your baby correctly at the breast. If you get mastitis more than once you should discuss your technique with a breastfeeding counsellor.

ENGORGEMENT

If the baby goes a long time between feeds, milk can collect in your breasts, making them hard and swollen. Engorgement can also occur if the baby is incorrectly positioned, even for just one feed. To treat it:

- Have a warm bath or shower, or apply warm flannels to the area, then express a little milk before latching your baby on. Be gentle: engorged breasts bruise easily.
- Do some arm swinging before feeding.
- Use a cold compress on the breast to reduce swelling.
- Feed frequently, or express if your baby won't oblige.
- Try drinking fennel or marigold tea three times a day.

It is important that you keep feeding if you suffer from any breast problems. It is quite safe to do so: any bacteria will be destroyed by acids in your baby's stomach.

Herbal teas may ease breastfeeding problems. A fennel or fenugreek seed infusion is said to enhance milk supply, while marigold tea may help with blocked ducts.

Common feeding problems

Most babies will quickly let you know if they have a problem with breastfeeding. They may cry during or after a feed, keep pulling off the breast or sometimes refuse point-blank to feed. This can be upsetting, but try not to take it as a personal rejection. Often there is a simple cause, which is commonly that the baby is not latching on properly. If it happens often and you can't work out why, a breastfeeding counsellor may be able to help. The following are all possible reasons for difficulty.

- If your breasts are engorged, your baby may find it hard to latch on. Express a little milk before the feed or hold a warm flannel against your breasts to help soften them a little.
- If your nipples are inverted or very flat, your baby may not be able to draw enough of the areola into his or her mouth (see box).
- Your milk flow may be so fast that it shocks the baby when he or she starts to suck. Try lying down or leaning well back (supported on lots of cushions) as you feed your baby. You can also try expressing a little milk just before the feed. Some women with a fast flow find that it helps to wear nipple shields while feeding.
- The baby may be frustrated when your milk flow slows down after the initial rush. Babies have to keep sucking in order to encourage more milk to be released from the production glands. If your baby stops feeding, it can help to switch to the other breast for a while before trying the first one again.
- Your milk supply may be low. There are several remedies you can try to enhance it (see below).

When breastfeeding goes well, it is deeply satisfying for mother and baby.

CORRECTING AN INVERTED NIPPLE
To help the baby grasp a flat or inverted nipple, take the areola between your thumb and first finger and gently press them together to push the nipple out. Then bring the baby towards you to latch on. Once the baby is attached, slowly release your fingers. Wearing breast shells between feeds can help to draw the nipples out.

- The baby may be windy. If your baby fusses halfway through a feed, he or she may need to be burped. Reflux, colic, teething or illness can also cause fussing.
- The baby may be distracted, particularly if he or she has just learned a new skill or if you are feeding in a noisy or unfamiliar place.
- You may have eaten or drunk something that the baby doesn't like.
- The baby may not be hungry. It's easy to get into the habit of nursing whenever your baby cries, but the problem may simply be that he or she is tired.

SLEEPY BABY

Some babies fall asleep after nursing for a few minutes, with the result that they need another feed very soon. This doesn't matter from time to time, but if it goes on you may want to encourage your baby to feed for longer.

- Make sure the baby is not too warm – feed in a cool room or remove a layer of clothing to help keep him or her awake.
- Rub the feet or walk your fingers up the back (either side of the spine) to keep the baby awake. Blow on his or her face, and stroke the cheek to stimulate the sucking reflex.
- Check that the baby's nose isn't squashed against your breast, since this can lead to sleepiness.
- Change the nappy halfway through a feed so that the baby is thoroughly awakened.

If your baby continues to be very sleepy and shows little interest in feeding, then he or she may be dehydrated or ill. See your doctor if you think this may be the case.

POOR WEIGHT GAIN

If your baby isn't gaining enough weight, don't be too quick to assume you can't make enough milk for his or her needs. A concerted effort to increase your milk flow can often solve the problem. Make sure you are getting

Left: It's hard to wake a sleepy baby. If you feel your baby has fallen asleep before they have enough, changing his or her nappy halfway through a feed will usually wake them up.

Right: There is not a lot you can do to prevent your baby from spitting up, but a cotton muslin will protect your clothes.

enough to drink and to eat – if you are dieting, it will be difficult for you to breastfeed. If you can, take your baby to bed with you for a couple of days; otherwise, spend as much time as possible together and feed frequently. Offer both breasts at each feed (starting on alternate ones each time). As with all breastfeeding problems, it is also worth checking your latching on, since if the baby is not attached to the breast in the right way he or she won't be able to empty it properly. Natural remedies for increasing milk supply include teas made from fennel, caraway or fenugreek seeds, nettle and blessed thistle. Certain foods such as oats and beans are also said to boost milk supply. In addition, it may be helpful to try to increase the fat content of your breastmilk by including more high-fat foods in your diet. Healthy options such as oily fish, nuts and avocados are best, but the odd bar of chocolate could help too.

SICKY BABY

Many breast- and bottle-fed babies bring up some milk after a feed, and some spit up quite a lot. This does not usually indicate a problem, so long as the baby is gaining weight normally, seems well and is producing wet nappies. But a baby who brings up part of a feed is likely to get hungry again quite soon. If the vomiting is frequent or forceful, the baby seems to be in pain or has watery stools, he or she needs to be seen by a doctor.

REFLUX

Some babies suffer from gastro-oesophageal reflux (heartburn). In this condition, the muscle at the entrance to the stomach doesn't close properly, which means that

stomach acid can travel back into the oesophagus. The baby often brings up large amounts of milk after feeding and may have poor weight gain. He or she may be distressed during and after every feed.

Try to keep your baby upright during and after feeds – use a sling and feed standing up, or try lying back against pillows and feeding so that the baby's tummy is against yours and he or she is facing the breast. Make sure you are both relaxed during feeds (breastfed babies tend to have less severe reflux at night when there is less distraction). Skin-to-skin contact, warmth and quiet will help. A homeopath may recommend the remedy Chamomilla or Nux vomica to ease discomfort. See your doctor if the symptoms persist.

Holding the baby so he or she is more vertical than horizontal can help babies with reflux or those who struggle with a fast milk flow. Leaning backwards may also help. Keep your baby's tummy against yours.

Deciding to bottle-feed

If you decide not to breastfeed, you will need to give your baby formula milk. Babies under the age of one can't have ordinary milk as their main drink because it contains too much salt and protein and not enough iron and other nutrients. Modern formula milks have been designed to resemble breastmilk as closely as possible. Most are based on cow's milk that has been modified to make it easier for babies to digest and to include the minerals and vitamins they need.

WHICH BABY MILK?

There is a huge range of baby milks on offer. Though there are not many differences between them, some do not contain added iron, which is recommended. If you want to use organic formula, the choice is easier because only a few brands are available.

There are two main types of formula: infant and follow-on. These have different ratios of the two main proteins in milk: whey and casein (curds). Infant milks are based on whey, which is more digestible. Follow-on milks are for babies of at least six months and contain more casein, which is denser and more satisfying. Some manufacturers also offer a casein-based milk for younger babies – often marketed as being for "the hungrier baby". It is best to start with an infant milk and to switch to a denser formula only if your baby seems to need it.

Formula milk is available in powdered form or ready-made in cartons. Ready-made milks are convenient if you are out and about, but they are expensive, so most

If you are going to bottle-feed your baby, then you will need to sterilize the bottles to prevent tummy upsets. An electric sterilizer does the job quickly.

When possible, give your baby skin-to-skin contact during a feed and concentrate on your baby to replicate the nursing experience.

people use powdered milk, which needs to be mixed with boiled water. Most organic milks are available only in powdered form, though this may change as they become more popular.

ALTERNATIVE FORMULAS

If your baby proves to be allergic to baby milk (see box), he or she may be able to tolerate a special cow's milk formula called protein hydrolysate formula. In this milk, the proteins have been broken down into smaller particles to make them easier to digest. Health professionals can advise you on this.

Another alternative is soy-based formula, the only vegan option. Soy-based formulas contain high levels of the plant chemical phytoestrogen, which can have an adverse effect on thyroid function, so you should not use them before discussing the implications with your doctor.

ALLERGIC TO FORMULA?
Signs of a true allergy include frequent diarrhoea, regular and forceful vomiting, excessive tiredness and skin rashes, but any of these symptoms should always be checked with a doctor since they may have other causes.

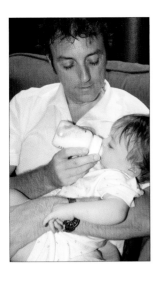

Left: Feeding time is a wonderful opportunity to sit quietly and cuddle your baby. Remember that sucking is a pleasure for the baby – concentrate on what you are doing together.

Right: Bottle-feeding allows the baby's father, or another person close to you to feed and bond with the baby.

Some parents prefer to give their baby a formula based on goat's milk, which can be easier to digest than cow's milk. However, it contains some of the same proteins, so a baby who is allergic to cow's milk formula may also react to goat's milk formula.

BONDING OVER A BOTTLE

Drinking milk is not only nourishing for your baby, it is pleasurable too. So take your time with feeding, and make it a loving and relaxing experience. When possible, loosen your baby's clothing and place him or her on your chest so that you are skin-to-skin. Look at and talk softly to your baby during the feed. It will help mother and baby to bond if she is the one to give most of the bottles for the first few weeks, with the father or one other close person lending a hand.

Make sure you are comfortable and put a pillow under the arm you are using to hold the baby. You will need to hold the baby slightly upright (at a 45-degree angle), with head well raised, so that the milk doesn't flow too fast. This will also help the baby to burp if necessary. To prevent the baby taking in too much air with the milk, hold the bottle up so that the teat is completely full. Never prop the bottle up and leave the baby to feed alone. Not only does this make feeding a rather lonely experience, it could lead to choking.

After the feed, help to release any air taken in with the milk by placing your baby against your shoulder and patting or rubbing the back until he or she burps. Sitting the baby on your lap, supporting the head with your hand or laying the baby on his or her tummy across your lap may also help. If any milk is left in the bottle you can keep it for up to an hour in case the baby wants more; after that it should be discarded.

HOW MUCH, HOW OFTEN?

Don't be in a hurry to put your baby on a feeding schedule. For the first few weeks, it is best to respond to the baby's needs and feed whenever he or she seems hungry. Babies' appetites vary and it will make both of you miserable if you restrict feeds or try to force the baby to accept more milk than he or she naturally takes. Offer the bottle whenever you think your baby wants it, and let him or her decide how much to drink – some babies will take a lot at one go and and then wait three to four hours before the next feed, others like to take less but feed more frequently. Over time, the gaps between feeds will get longer and you'll be able to plan your day around your baby's natural feeding pattern.

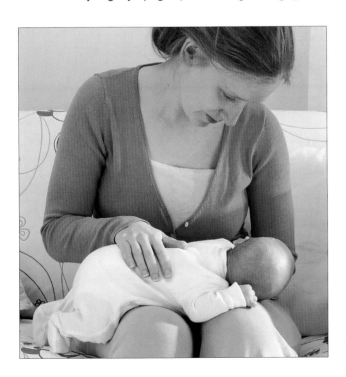

Experiment to find the best way of winding your baby. Try laying the baby across your lap, keeping the head slightly higher than his or her body.

Bottle-feeding basics

You will need at least six bottles and teats. You can reuse another baby's bottles, so long as they are not scratched, but you should always buy new teats, and there are lots of different ones on the market. Teats have different flow rates: slow, medium and fast. Generally, if your baby empties the bottle in just a few minutes, the flow rate may be too fast; if the feed takes half an hour or longer, the flow rate may be too slow.

If your bottles have wide necks, you can mix up the feed in them. If not, you will need a measuring jug and a plastic fork or knife (of a type that can be sterilized) for mixing the formula. You'll also need a bottlebrush and sterilizing equipment.

KEEPING CLEAN

Bacteria multiply quickly in milk, so it is vital that any bottles you use are scrupulously clean and sterilized to protect your baby from gastroenteritis and tummy upsets. Always wash bottles in hot water and washing-up liquid, and use a bottlebrush to clean around the rim of the bottle and the screw top. Squeeze washing-up liquid into the teat and use your fingers to clean it, turning it inside out to ensure that no residue remains. Rinse in hot water and then sterilize.

You should always wash your hands with soap and water before giving your baby a feed, and before making up the milk. Don't keep milk at room temperature for more than an hour or so, and always throw away any milk left over at the end of a feed.

Always keep bottles of formula in the refrigerator once you have made them up. It is important to keep them cold to prevent bacteria from multiplying. If you haven't used the bottles within 24 hours, discard the milk.

WHICH STERILIZING METHOD?

Steam sterilizer units are the easiest and quickest way to sterilize feeding equipment, and don't use any chemicals. You simply add a little water, close the lid and switch on.

Boiling needs no special equipment except a large, lidded pan, which you should keep just for sterilizing. Fill with cold water, add the bottles and lids and submerge completely (making sure that no air is trapped in them), then boil for ten minutes with the lid on. Don't take the lid off until you need the equipment: once you remove the lid the water is no longer sterile, so you must take everything out (wash your hands before doing this).

Chemical sterilizing can be a useful method if you are away from home, but it is probably too time-consuming for general use. You can buy a cold-water sterilizing unit or use any large container, such as a bucket, with a lid. You will also need sterilizing solution or tablets. Make up the solution according to the manufacturer's instructions, and add to the bucket. Immerse the bottles, lids and teats

Before you embark on bottle-feeding, you need to have all the necessary equipment, including enough bottles to see you through 24 hours, a bottle brush, measuring jug, and plastic cutlery that can be sterilized.

Many plastic baby bottles are made from polycarbonate plastic, which contains the hormone-disrupting chemical Bisphenol A. Minute amounts of this chemical may leak into the baby's milk, especially when the bottle is heated, or if the surface is scratched. Although the risks are very small, as a precaution you may want to buy bottles made from heat-resistant toughened glass (which can also be recycled) or from polypropylene plastic, which does not contain Bisphenol A. Check on the internet for manufacturers of suitable brands.

Some babies don't mind drinking milk cold, but most prefer it to be the same temperature as breastmilk.

completely (making sure that no air is trapped in them) and use a plate to weigh them down. Leave for at least two hours, or as specified by the chemical manufacturer. Wash your hands before taking out the bottles. If you want to rinse off the chemical solution, use boiled, cooled water, not tap water (which isn't sterile).

When your baby is ready for a feed, take the bottle from the fridge and heat in a bowl of hot water, keeping it out of children's reach. Shake the bottle, then test the temperature with a few drops on your wrist.

Making up a feed

You can make up each feed as you need it, but it will save time if you prepare all the bottles your baby will need for 24 hours in one go. It also means that if you've got a furiously hungry baby you have the vital feed ready at hand.

Put the caps on the bottles and store them in the fridge until required. Make sure everything you use for making up the feed – bottles, tops, teats, measuring jug, plastic knife and fork – is clean and sterile.

1 Always use freshly boiled water: empty the kettle, rinse it and fill with cold water. Boil, then leave it to cool. Wash your hands. Pour the correct amount of water into a measuring jug, or directly into bottles.

2 Add the exact number of scoops of formula recommended by the manufacturer (usually, one level scoop per 30ml/1fl oz water). Overfill the scoop and then level off the powder using the back of a sterile knife. Do not pack the powder down.

3 If you are using a jug, stir with a fork to mix, then pour the formula into the bottles. If you are mixing in the bottle, add the teat, the disc and the cap and shake well to mix. When all the bottles are full, put them in the centre of the fridge so they chill quickly.

4 Before a feed, warm the milk in a bowl of hot (not boiling) water. Don't use a microwave oven, which heats unevenly and can cause hot spots. Test it is at blood temperature by shaking a few drops on to your wrist; it should feel neither hot nor cold.

Crying, responding and sleeping

❝ As babies get older they are more interested in noise, colour and movement, and will respond to your efforts to entertain them. **❞**

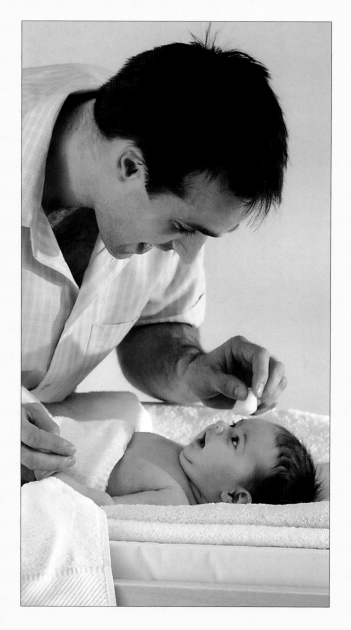

It's normal for babies to cry. It is the only way that they can communicate with us, to let us know when they are hungry, cold, uncomfortable or lonely. But some babies definitely cry more than others. A British study, conducted in Manchester, found that the amount young babies cried over the course of a day could be as little as a few minutes or as much as five hours.

Many babies are naturally easy-going. They cry only for obvious reasons, such as hunger or when they are startled. They may also be easy to soothe, once you have worked out what they like best: being rocked or sung to perhaps.

If your baby cries a lot, it is very easy to feel that you are doing something wrong. It is true that there is sometimes a clear cause for frequent crying, such as illness or persistent hunger, which obviously needs to be addressed. But often babies who cry a lot are highly sensitive, and simply find it hard to cope with all the stimuli that they are bombarded with in a normal day. If this is the case with your

There is no doubt that some babies are easier to care for than others. If you have a high-need baby, the calm moments can be all the more special.

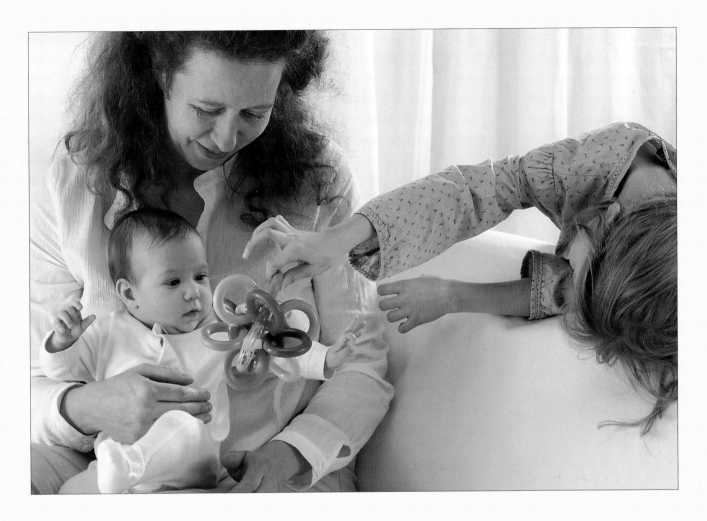

baby, you will have to call on all your reserves of compassion and patience to nurture him or her through this tricky stage. It can be very helpful to remember that it won't go on forever: sensitive babies often settle down after three or four months. This is also the time when you can expect your baby's sleep pattern to begin to coincide more with yours. Very young babies don't distinguish between night and day and, if anything, they tend to be more wakeful at night.

There is a lot you can do to help your baby sleep better right from the start. But, like so many aspects of parenting, having a relaxed attitude and realistic expectations is important and will help you to cope with the inevitable disturbances and disruptions to your painstakingly established routines.

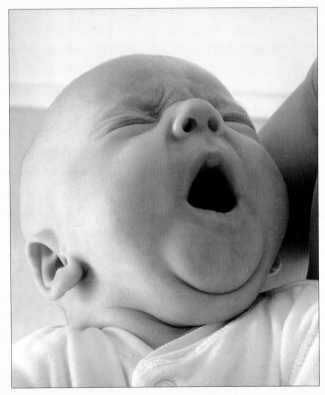

Top: As babies get older they become more interested in noise, colour and movement, and will start to respond to your efforts to entertain them.

Babies have all sorts of new things to look at and experience in a day. It's not surprising that they can become overwhelmed in these early months.

Why babies cry

Crying is the only way a very young baby can communicate. And it is a very effective method for the baby to get attention: when you rush to soothe your crying baby, you are doing what comes naturally to parents all over the world. Babies cry in different ways depending on what is wrong. In time you will learn to distinguish between cries, and recognize the different sounds your baby makes when hungry, uncomfortable or overtired. You may also start to pick up on certain gestures – for example, arching the back when windy – or you may become more aware of what triggers your baby's distress – such as too much handling by visitors.

CHECKLIST: WHY IS MY BABY CRYING?

In the early days, discovering why your baby is crying is a matter of trial and error. It's helpful to have a mental checklist of possible causes that you can run through to help you pinpoint the cause.

Is the baby hungry? Young babies can get hungry more quickly than you would think possible. They go through growth spurts, which means they suddenly need to feed more than usual. So even if you have fed your baby very recently, crying may mean he or she is hungry.

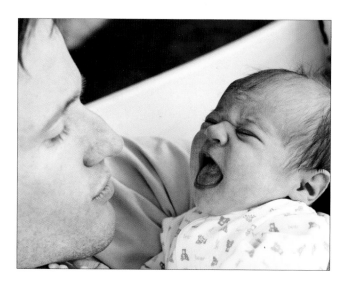

Don't worry that you are teaching your baby bad habits by attending to his or her cries. You are showing that you can be relied on to be there when needed.

Is the baby wet? Some infants hate feeling wet, and will scream when their nappy is dirty or a cloth nappy is damp. Others don't mind it at all.

Is the baby uncomfortable? Babies cry if they are too hot or cold, if their clothing is tight or uncomfortable, and sometimes when they are having a bowel movement. Check that the room is warm enough and that your baby is dressed appropriately. Make sure that clothing isn't rubbing, scratching or pressing against the skin. Check fingers and toes, too – perhaps a hair is wound tightly around a tiny digit. Have a look at the nappy (diaper) area – the cause may be a painful rash.

Has the baby been startled? New babies often jerk around a lot, especially when they are dropping off to sleep. A baby who is frightened – by a loud noise, say – will cry. All the baby needs is to be held close until he or she calms down. Swaddling or holding close can help your baby to feel secure and prevent any sudden movements that will be disturbing.

Does the baby dislike being naked? Some babies cry whenever they are changed or washed. If this is the case with yours, be as quick and gentle as you can. Laying a small towel over a naked baby's chest and tummy may help him or her feel more secure. Making eye contact, talking and singing may also be reassuring.

At difficult moments, focus on calming yourself down – if you are tense, you will find it harder to soothe your baby. Relax your shoulders and breathe slowly.

Has the baby got wind? Babies cry during or after a feed if they need burping, and some may need burping again later on when the milk is being digested. Sometimes they need to pass wind: it can help your baby to do this if you pat his or her bottom rhythmically. Your breastfed baby may also cry if you have eaten a particular food that he or she is sensitive to.

Is the baby ill? Babies who are crying in a different way than usual may be unwell. Check the baby over: is there a rash, a temperature, a runny nose or other signs of illness? Call a doctor if your baby is crying strangely or persistently, or looks or behaves unusually.

Is the baby overstimulated? Babies can become irritable if they get too much stimulation; they cry as a way of shutting out external noise. If your baby is tired and overstimulated, he or she will find it hard to drop off.

You will soon learn how to comfort your baby: some like to be held upright, others prefer being cradled.

Being held, rocked, or patted on the back is a good way to settle an overtired baby, but some seem to prefer being laid down in a quiet, dark place and allowed to cry for a minute or two, after which they will go to sleep.

Is the baby lonely? Babies need lots of physical contact, and will cry if they want to be picked up and cuddled. If you find it hard to hold your baby as much as he or she seems to want, take it in turns with a partner, enlist the help of a grandparent or friend, or use a sling to carry the baby while keeping your hands free.

You will often hear parents say that they are happy to leave their babies to cry so long as they know they are fed, burped and changed. But a baby may be crying simply because he or she feels fearful or lonely and needs your comforting presence.

AM I SPOILING MY BABY?

Young babies are not capable of crying in order to manipulate you – their brains don't work that way. They cry because they have a need that isn't being met; making a noise is the only way that they can signal that something is wrong. It's important that your baby learns he or she is safe and can rely on you. Don't hesitate to pick the baby up for a cuddle whenever he or she is upset. In this way, you help to establish a relationship based on trust and love.

Researchers have found that the more quickly their carers respond to their cries, the more quickly and easily babies are soothed. In other words, if you leave your baby to cry for ten minutes in the hope that he or she will settle, it may take you much longer to calm him or her down. Other studies show that babies whose cries are quickly and consistently responded to in the first months will develop into more independent toddlers than those who are often left to cry. So don't worry that you are teaching your baby bad habits by attending to his or her cries. You are letting the baby know that you can be relied on to be there when you are needed.

Soothing your baby

If your baby is crying, check the basics first: offer a feed and check for a wet or dirty nappy. Try burping to release any trapped air. If your baby is clean, fed and burped, but still crying, one or a combination of the following methods may be soothing.

GETTING PHYSICAL

Bear in mind that no one method works for all babies – finding out what calms your baby is a matter of experimentation, and nothing will work every time.

Hold the baby close. Physical contact has a calming effect, especially if you place your baby naked on your bare skin. Try shutting out any other stimuli by going into a dark, warm room. You may find that changing the way you hold the baby is also soothing – try an upright position or the colic hold (see Coping with Colic).

Try rocking. Most babies love to be swayed from side to side – it's the same movement they experienced in the womb. Researchers have found that parents automatically rock their children approximately in time with a heartbeat. If rocking doesn't seem to work for your baby, try upping the tempo a little – about 60 rocks a minute is good. Rocking your baby in a pram can also be very soothing, or you can use a sling and walk around.

Dance. If your baby is agitated, playing music or singing while you dance rhythmically with the baby in your arms

may help to soothe him or her. You can gradually slow the pace as the crying subsides.

Let the baby suck on something. Some babies are very "sucky" and like to nurse for comfort for long periods. If you are not breastfeeding – or if you are but your baby doesn't seem to want the breast – your clean little finger makes an excellent temporary pacifier. Dummies can also work well or you can try guiding your baby's own fingers to his or her mouth to suck on.

Keep the baby warm. A baby who feels warm and cosy may calm down more quickly. Heat the room to a comfortable temperature and wrap your baby in blankets or try swaddling (see Coping with Colic).

GOOD NOISE

Before birth, babies are exposed to constant noise from their mother's heartbeat, her muted voice and the low rumble of the womb. So similar kinds of noise can be comforting for distressed infants.

Left: Shushing helps to shut out extraneous noise and also relaxes the baby as it recalls the noise of the womb. This is why we instinctively use this sound to soothe babies.

Right: Holding your baby close for a while may be soothing, but you may also need to rock a crying baby, or offer your little finger to suck.

Left: Babies have been seen sucking a thumb in the womb – it is a great way of self-soothing.

Right: Long bouts of crying are rare in cultures where babies are carried all day, so it may just be that your crying baby wants to be held. Using a sling and more cuddling or nursing may reduce your baby's crying.

Shush. Shushing is a traditional and effective way to quieten a baby – simply place your mouth a little distance from your baby's ear and say "sssssshhhhhh". Do long shushes, increasing the volume if your baby doesn't seem to be responding.

Sing. The other sound traditionally used to soothe a baby is singing. It doesn't matter whether you have a good voice or not – your baby will appreciate your singing. It's worth learning a couple of lullabies for this purpose.

Use white noise. The roar of a vacuum cleaner, the hum of a washing machine or untuned radio static can all quieten a baby, sometimes in an instant. You can buy CDs of these sounds or record your own. It's not a good idea to operate a vacuum cleaner near your baby for long periods since this will affect the quality of the air that he or she is breathing.

Play music. Classical music has been shown to have a soothing effect on babies, and Mozart has been shown to be particularly good (no one knows why). But try light concertos rather than, say, operas.

CHANGE THE ENVIRONMENT

Consider your surroundings. If it is noisy and bright, with lots of activity, the baby may feel overwhelmed.

Take the baby somewhere quieter. Sometimes a change of place is all a baby needs to calm down.

Get some fresh air. Going outdoors will often stop a baby crying – and it can help you to relax too. Many babies fall asleep when driven around in a car for a while, even if they wake up the instant you stop the car.

Pass the baby to somebody else. If you haven't been able to soothe your baby, ask your partner or another close person to take a turn. Don't take it personally if the crying stops – it may just be that the change of company has distracted the baby.

A crying baby may be distracted from his or her distress by something new – an interesting toy, a funny noise or even a comical expression.

Try diversion. Offer a toy, walk in front of a mirror so that the baby can see his or her reflection, or walk around the house. Some babies find a warm bath very soothing; others don't.

AND FINALLY...

If all else fails, just stop trying to calm your baby down and accept the fact that for some reason he or she needs to cry. Continue to hold the baby close, but make a positive effort to release any tension that you might be feeling. Let your shoulders drop downward, take a long slow breath in and then out. Sit quietly for a few minutes, holding your crying child, controlling your breathing, and allowing yourself to accept the difficulty of the situation. If you can be relaxed about what is happening, you may well find that the baby stops crying in response.

Baby massage routine

Massage is a wonderful way to build a loving bond of trust between parent and child, and can be a useful part of a bedtime routine. It has practical benefits, too: it can stimulate your baby's circulation and immature immune system, and it helps to improve the digestion. Massage is best done when your baby is already relaxed and calm, so aim to do it between feeds – a massage may be uncomfortable immediately after feeding, and if the baby is hungry he or she won't want to lie still. Don't try to do anything else, like watch TV, while you are

WHEN NOT TO MASSAGE
Check with your doctor or health adviser if your baby has health problems or if you have any doubts about the suitability of massage. Do not massage if your baby is ill or has a skin condition, and wait for 48 hours after immunization – longer if the baby has been adversely affected. Stop the massage if your baby doesn't enjoy it, and drop or adapt any movements that he or she does not seem to like.

As your baby grows and becomes more robust, you can increase the pressure slightly, but never be firm or probing. Newborns should simply be gently stroked.

massaging your baby – make this a quiet and precious time that you can both enjoy: go to a quiet place and switch off any bright overhead lights. As you massage, keep looking at your baby – smiling, chatting and singing will help to maintain his or her interest.

Massage techniques

You can massage your baby clothed or naked. A naked massage gives the skin-to-skin contact that babies enjoy, but use oil so your hands glide over the skin without pulling. An ordinary vegetable oil such as olive or sunflower is ideal. Make sure that the room is warm, and lay your baby on a thick towel so that he or she is comfortable (you can place a clean nappy under a naked baby). Take a few slow breaths to help you relax. Use light strokes that are just firm enough not to be ticklish – this routine is for babies of about one month or older. Do each stroke several times.

1 Lay your baby on his or her back and look into his or her eyes. Place your palms together and gently lay the sides of your little fingers on the centre of the baby's chest. Slowly open your hands, keeping the thumbs together and sliding the little fingers apart until your hands are flat on the baby's body. Stay like this for a few moments.

2 Tell your baby you are going to give him or her a massage. Slowly stroke down the baby's torso. Start by using both hands then turn your hand so that it covers the top of the baby's chest. Gently stroke down the torso. As you do so, place your other hand at the top of the baby's chest. Stroke one hand after the other in a smooth action.

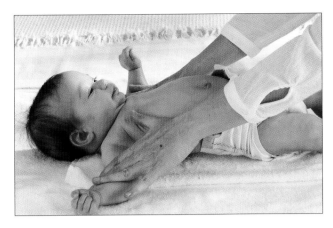

3 Rest your hands on the baby's chest and stroke upwards and outwards so that your hands pass down the baby's arms and hands.

4 Now stroke both hands all the way down the torso, gradually lengthening the strokes to include the baby's legs. Take the left leg in one hand, using the other to support the ankle. Work your way down the leg using a gentle squeezing action.

5 Take the left foot in your hand, supporting the heel with one hand. Use the thumb of your other hand to stroke over the sole, from the inner to the outer edge, and from the heel to the toe. Do the same on the right foot.

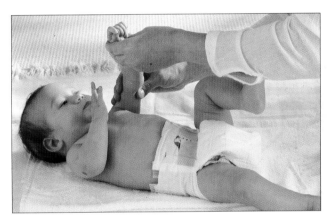

6 Now take the left arm in one hand, holding the baby's hand or wrist with your other hand. Work down the arm to the wrist, gently squeezing, then change hands so that you maintain a continuous action. Do the same on the right arm.

7 Gently rest your hand on the baby's abdomen and trace an arch from the bottom right of the trunk to the bottom left – this follows the digestive path. Take care not to press down.

8 Turn your baby over, remove the nappy if you want to. Place your hands over the shoulder blades and draw your hands all the way down the spine and over the back of the legs. Using the flat of your hand, trace an arch from the right buttock to the left one, then stroke down the back of the body again.

Coping with colic

A young baby who has regular and long bouts of inconsolable crying with no apparent cause is said to have colic. About one in five babies are affected. Nobody knows exactly what colic is or what causes it, but there are many theories. In a few cases, it may be caused by a cow's milk intolerance or, in breastfed babies, by a reaction to something in the mother's diet. The crying could also be due to discomfort from reflux or wind. However, in many cases, colic may simply be a sensitive baby's reaction to all the stimulation received during the day. The immature nervous system becomes overloaded and the baby expresses this through crying.

Colic is hard for parents to cope with, but it is important to remember that it does stop in time. Try to arrange for help at the time of day when your baby is likely to cry. If you find the crying unbearable, don't hesitate to get support: your doctor or health visitor should be sympathetic, or you can call a voluntary organisation such as Cry-sis. Remember that you can place the baby in a safe place – such as the cot – and go into another room if you need a breather.

IS IT COLIC?
Colic usually starts when a baby is two to four weeks old and lasts for up to four months. Babies are said to have colic when:
• they have lengthy bouts of crying on most days
• there is no obvious cause

Many colicky babies:
• have crying bouts at the same time each day, usually in the late afternoon or evening
• draw their knees up to their chest and clench their fists, as if they are in pain, and are red in the face
• may pass wind or have difficulty passing stools

A small study of 28 babies found that cranial osteopathy reduced crying and improved sleep in colicky babies.

SOOTHING A COLICKY BABY
Reduce external stimuli – turn off overhead lights, music and the television. Then try doing all of the following, one after the other, or use the techniques separately.
• Swaddle your baby in a light blanket or shawl (see box)
• Hold the baby close so that you place gentle pressure on the abdomen: hold the baby along your forearm in the colic hold (see picture)
• Shush in the baby's ear or play white noise.
• Rock the baby in your arms.
• Give the baby something to suck on, such as your little finger or a dummy (pacifier).

USING A DUMMY OR PACIFIER
Babies love to suck. You can sometimes encourage a baby to suck on his or her own fingers or thumb by guiding them to the mouth. Alternatively you can give the baby a dummy (pacifier), which, used wisely, is useful if your baby needs to suck a lot.
• Never dip a dummy in sugar or honey.
• Don't use a string or ribbon to tie a dummy around the baby's neck.
• Don't use a dummy in the first six weeks if you are breastfeeding.
• Don't give your baby a dummy whenever he or she is upset (it will become a hard-to-break habit).
• Ideally, restrict use to sleep times and colic.
• Wash and sterilize dummies between each use.
• Throw a dummy away if it shows signs of damage.

SWADDLING YOUR BABY

Some babies prefer to be wrapped so their arms and hands are free. You will need a stretchy, light blanket or cotton sheet about 90cm/3ft square.

1 Place the sheet diagonally on a flat surface and fold down the top corner by about 15cm/6in. Place the baby so that his or her neck rests on the folded edge.

2 Straighten the baby's arm at the side, then pull one side of the blanket over the arm and across the body. Tuck it under the back at the opposite side.

3 Fold the bottom of the sheet over the feet and the baby's body. Tuck it into the first fold to secure it. Straighten the free arm, then pull the other side of the sheet over it and across the baby's body, as in step 2. Tuck it under the back on the opposite side.

WORTH A TRY?

One common over-the-counter remedy is simethicone. However, studies have shown it to be no more effective than a placebo. The following are proven to help some infants with colic, so may be worth trying with your baby.

- If you are bottle-feeding and think your baby may be allergic to formula, ask your doctor about using a hypoallergenic formula.
- If you are breastfeeding, take note of what you eat and see if certain foods seem to make your baby's colic worse. Tea, coffee and colas, dairy products, alcohol, spicy foods, citrus fruits, onions, garlic, cabbage, broccoli and cauliflower may all have an effect. If you notice a correlation, cut out the offending food for a few days to see if your baby cries less. If you cut out dairy products, make sure you get enough calcium from other food sources or a supplement.
- Consider taking your baby to a cranial osteopath for treatment. Sometimes the pressure of the delivery can cause slight misalignments in the way the flat bones of the skull join together, causing headaches and distress. A cranial osteopath will very gently manipulate the bones to relieve any pressure, and this can sometimes have a miraculous effect on a previously colicky baby.

Many hospitals advise against swaddling at night because of the risk of overheating, but wrapping can be very soothing when you are awake and can keep an eye on your baby.

Some parents can't imagine life without dummies, others think they are an abomination. But, used wisely, they are useful if you have a baby who wants to comfort-suck a lot.

- To prevent wind and help with reflux, feed in an upright position and make sure you burp after every feed. If you are breastfeeding, get an expert to check your technique. If bottle-feeding, try using a teat with bigger holes; if they are too small, your baby may be swallowing lots of air with the milk.

For the colic hold, support the baby's crotch with your hand while the tummy rests on your forearm and the head is near your elbow. For the reverse colic hold, support the head with your hand; the baby's front rests on your forearm and the crotch on your elbow.

Cool, diluted chamomile or fennel tea can help to soothe a gripy tummy. Be very wary of other herbal remedies for colic – star anise used to be recommended but it has caused poisoning in some infants.

A place to sleep

Young babies sleep when they are tired, and they stay asleep as long as they need to. It doesn't matter to them whether they are in a cot or being carried through a crowded shopping centre. If your baby needs sleep, he or she will drop off without your help.

It is inevitable that your baby will fall asleep often when you are holding him or her, and cuddling a sleeping newborn is one of the silent joys of parenthood. But if this happens every time, your baby will associate sleeping with being held. As a rule, it is a good idea to put babies down when they are looking tired or yawning so that they learn to drop off in bed. It's impossible to do this all the time, especially if you are breastfeeding. But letting your baby fall asleep on his or her own sometimes will help establish good sleep patterns for the future.

If your baby protests at being put down, try stroking or patting him or her in the cot. Singing or playing soothing music can also help the baby to relax. A musical mobile can distract and lull the baby to sleep.

Putting your baby to sleep on his or her back is the best way to reduce the risk of SIDS. Some babies don't like this, but they will get used to it in time if you always put them on their backs. However, if you decide to let your baby sleep on one side, make sure the lower arm is to the front to prevent the baby from rolling forward.

CHECKLIST: SAFE SLEEP

All parents worry about their babies, and most find themselves checking on sleeping infants from time to time. The following steps reduce the risk of a baby suffering SIDS (sudden infant death syndrome).

- Always put your baby to sleep on his or her back.
- Put your baby to sleep on a firm mattress (not a sheepskin or pillow).
- Do not let anyone smoke near your baby (if possible, ban smoking from your home).
- Do not let your baby get too hot (or too cold) – keep the room temperature comfortable. Never put the cot next to a radiator or heater, or let your baby sleep with a hot-water bottle or electric blanket.
- Put the baby's feet at the base of the cot (the feet-to-foot position) so that he or she cannot wriggle down under the covers.
- Keep the baby's head uncovered. Make sure that covers reach no higher than the shoulders and are tucked in securely.
- Use sheets and thin blankets only (cellular blankets are ideal). Don't use duvets, pillows, wedges or bedding rolls.
- Don't use plastic sheets, cot bumpers or anything with strings or ribbons in your baby's bed. Keep toys out of the cot when your baby is sleeping.
- Seek medical advice promptly if your baby is ill.

A SNUG BED

Some babies happily sleep in a cot from birth, but most seem to prefer being in a cosier space (which is what, after all, they have been used to in the womb). A Moses basket, rocking crib or the carrycot from a pram are all suitable, and your baby can sleep in one until he or she gets too big for it, or is starting to roll over.

Your baby's mattress should be firm and clean – it is best to buy a new one for each baby. Choose one with a removable, washable waterproof covering or a complete PVC covering, and clean and air it regularly. Check that it fits well – there shouldn't be any gaps between the edges of the mattress and the sides of the cot.

A PLACE FOR NAPS

Opinions vary on whether it is best for your baby to be in the same place for every sleep, or whether it is helpful to differentiate between daytime naps and nighttime sleeping. Like many aspects of baby

You don't need a baby monitor unless your baby's room is out of earshot. If you do get a monitor, choose one that monitors sound only – a breathing monitor can just increase your anxiety levels, which is counterproductive.

There is no need to keep everyone quiet while your baby naps. Young babies can sleep through normal household noise, and it is a good idea to get them used to this from the beginning.

care, it is down to what suits you and your baby best. You will probably find it easier to go out and about if your baby takes daytime naps in a pram. But some babies settle better when they are placed in their own cot in a darkened room. Experiment to see what works for you.

SLEEPING WITH YOUR BABY

It is recommended that your baby should share your room for at least six months. A baby who sleeps near his or her mother may be better able to regulate breathing. However, it is best for a young baby to sleep in a cot. An adult bed is not designed for a baby, who could become trapped between the mattress and headboard, or suffocate if a sleeping adult rolls on him or her.

Although a cot is the safest place for a baby to sleep, many mothers find that they do end up sharing their bed with their baby for part or all of the night. Bedsharing also makes breastfeeding easier – women who co-sleep tend to breastfeed for longer. A bedside cot can give you the best of both worlds. But ultimately you will make your own decision about what is right for you and your baby. If you decide to bedshare, there are some extra safety precautions you need to take into account.

WHEN NOT TO SLEEP WITH YOUR BABY

It may be inadvisable to bedshare with a premature or small-at-birth baby or a baby with a fever.
Never sleep with your baby:
- If you smoke.
- If you have drunk alcohol or taken drugs, or if you are ill or so tired that you may find it hard to respond to your baby.
- On a sofa or armchair.

Even if you don't sleep with your baby, you'll certainly enjoy spending time on your bed together.

- Sleep on a firm, flat mattress – not a sofa, armchair, waterbed, beanbag or soft and sagging mattress.
- Do not place the baby between you and your partner – fathers are less aware of their babies and so may be more likely to roll on top of them.
- Make sure that your baby cannot fall out of bed or be wedged between the side of the mattress and the wall. A guard rail is useful.
- Dress your baby in no more clothing than you would wear in bed yourself. Use lightweight covers for your baby, not the duvet.
- Make sure that the covers cannot cover the baby's head and that he or she can't wriggle under a pillow.
- Don't leave the baby alone in the bed.

If you have twins, you may like to put them in the same cot. A study by the University of Durham showed that putting twins in the same sleeping space was safe, provided all the safe sleep guidelines were followed.

How babies sleep

Babies spend a lot of their time asleep, but they don't go about it in a way that is convenient for their parents. Small babies have lots of naps – an hour here, two or three there. This is because they have tiny stomachs and need feeding frequently. Bottle-fed babies tend to go longer than breastfed babies because formula milk takes longer to digest.

Unlike adults, young babies don't operate on a 24-hour cycle, and they don't distinguish between day and night. In the early weeks, there is very little you can do about this. So there is little point in trying to establish a sleep routine early on.

Gradually, your baby will adapt to the daily rhythm of light and dark. By the age of three or four months, most babies are sleeping about twice as much at night as during the day. Some babies may even sleep through the night at this stage, but most still wake up at least once a night to feed.

BABIES' SLEEP CYCLES
Like adults, babies sleep in cycles of active (dream) sleep and quiet sleep. A baby is more likely to wake at the end of one of these cycles, which usually last between 45 minutes and an hour. An adult cycle lasts up to two hours, but we usually don't remember waking up because we have learned ways of putting ourselves straight back to sleep.

A good feed at bedtime will help to lull your baby into a long and restful sleep.

CREATING A GOOD SLEEPING ENVIRONMENT
You can encourage a young baby to get as much sleep as possible at night by providing a good sleeping environment for them.
- Keep the room warm (16–18°C/60–65°F). Make sure that your baby's cot isn't positioned in a draught.
- Darken the room. Use a low lamp to tend to your baby at night.
- Position the cot somewhere quiet. If it is near a window, outside noises may wake your baby up.
- Change your baby at night only when it's really necessary. Even then, keep activity to a minimum – speak as little as possible and only in a low voice.
- Similarly, make night feeds quiet and functional.

STRUCTURING THE DAY
Giving a baby a good daytime routine can help to improve nighttime sleep. If your baby tends to sleep late to make up for a restless night, try waking him or her up earlier to help the baby's body clock adjust to yours. Prioritize daytime sleep even if it means missing out on some activities or going for long walks in order to get your baby to drop off.

Young babies nap several times a day. Once they reach the age of three or four months, and start sleeping longer at night, they have longer periods of wakefulness during

The average newborn sleeps for about 16 hours a day – but yours may not need this much sleep, or may sleep much longer. Some babies get by on as little as eight hours a day.

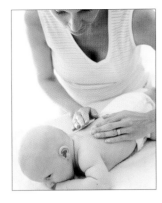

A set bedtime routine might be a warm bath, then being dressed before you do any final winding-down activities such as a feed.

A very gentle, soothing massage might be what your baby enjoys as part of the bedtime routine, but only if he or she finds it soothing.

Babies need a quiet room to sleep in without too much stimulus. Keep toys hidden in cupboards and out of the cot, so that there is nothing to distract them from sleep.

the day. But they still need at least two naps. It is important to realize that babies get tired very quickly. Most need a nap about two hours after they wake up, and another longer nap in the early afternoon. So if they wake up at 7.00 am, they will need a sleep around 9.00 am and again at about midday. Young babies also need another sleep in the late afternoon (as may some older babies). It is best if this nap is kept short, though, or nighttime sleep will be affected. It's helpful to put your baby down for a sleep after a feed, which has a naturally soporific effect. Don't restrict daytime sleep in the hope that your baby will sleep better at night – it is likely to have the opposite effect. An overtired baby is likely to sleep fitfully at night.

Some babies take only short naps. If this is the case for yours, it may be worth noting the times when the baby wakes after first dropping off. Then try going to the cot a few minutes before the usual wake-up time and stroking or singing your baby back to sleep if there are signs of stirring. This may help the baby to sleep for longer, and eventually he or she should do this without you going in.

Schedule plenty of activity in the afternoon, then have extended calm-down time in the run up to bedtime. Most importantly, feed regularly. Some older babies are hard to feed during the day because they are distracted – and they then need to feed more at night. Feeding in a dark, quiet room can help them to concentrate.

A GOOD BEDTIME ROUTINE

Babies respond well to repetition, and an evening routine can help your baby to settle well at night. Three or four months is a good age to institute a bedtime routine, but you can start it earlier if you like. Try to stop boisterous play (such as tickling) at least an hour or so before the

Give your baby plenty of kick-around time. An active day can help a baby to sleep better at night.

baby's bedtime. Make this a quiet wind-down time, with gentle play. Your bedtime routine could include some of the following. It will help if you stick to the same elements in the same order each evening. But don't make a bedtime routine too complicated or it will take you ages to put your baby to bed.

- Warm bath
- Massage
- Being dressed in nightclothes
- Story or song
- Lights out
- Breastfeed or bottle
- Kiss and cuddle
- Time alone in the cot, perhaps with a musical mobile, a ticking clock, radio turned down low or a CD of lullabies to help lull the baby to sleep.

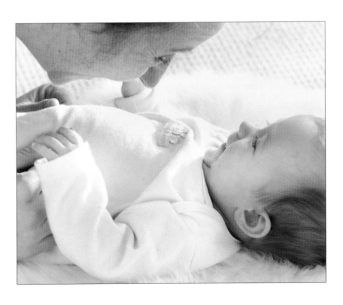

Helping a wakeful baby sleep

Most parents want their children to sleep through the night, but it is important to realize that in the early months most babies are unable to sleep for longer than five hours at a stretch. If your young baby goes from midnight to 5.00 am without waking, you can consider that to be sleeping through the night. By the end of the first year, your baby may sleep for 10–12 hours at a stretch. But many babies continue to wake up at least once at night. All babies will have wakeful periods from time to time, especially if they are teething or ill.

IMPROVING SLEEP

If your baby is still waking up several times a night after the age of three or four months, it may be that something is preventing him or her from sleeping longer. It is worth going through the following checklist to see if you can encourage a better sleeping pattern.

Is your baby getting enough fresh air? Research shows that babies who go out in daylight after 2.00 pm get a better night's sleep.

Is your baby having enough daytime naps? If a baby doesn't sleep much during the day, he or she may well have more disturbed sleep at night.

Is he or she sleeping too much during the day? Don't let your baby sleep for more than three hours at a time during the day, or night sleep may be affected. Keep naps in the late afternoon to no more than 30 minutes.

Is he or she getting enough stimulation? It is important to let your baby have a good kick-around on the floor and for you to provide new experiences to enjoy. Babies tend to be most alert in the afternoon and early evening, so this is a good time to take them out.

Make sure your baby has plenty of opportunity for stimulation and movement during the day.

A study of English babies in 2003 found that fewer than a quarter of them were sleeping through the night by the age of ten months.

COMFORTERS

If your baby wakes in the night a comforter can help him or her get back to sleep. Provide the same soft toy or piece of cloth every time the baby goes to sleep. It will help if you imbue it with your scent – place it between you and the baby every time you breastfeed, or wear it next to your skin for a day or two. If your baby takes to the comforter, make sure you have at least one spare for when it is in the wash or in case it gets lost.

Is he or she getting too much stimulation? If your baby is being distracted when he or she is getting sleepy, it may be harder to drop off at night. Be alert to signs of tiredness: yawning, turning the head away, rubbing eyes.

Is he or she getting enough milk? A hungry baby may often be lulled back to sleep temporarily but will keep waking up until he or she is given milk. Both bottle-fed and breast-fed babies benefit from being given a feed at about 10.00 pm, or at the parents' bedtime, to help them sleep through the main part of the night.

Is bedtime early enough? Most babies like to go to sleep at 6.30–7.30 pm. If yours is getting to bed much later, try putting him or her to sleep 15 minutes earlier each evening until you reach this time.

Is the baby warm enough? If a baby is too cold, he or she will wake up. A baby sleeping bag is good if covers tend to be kicked off.

Is the room too light? Invest in blackout blinds if light from the street or the sun is waking your baby up.

Are your expectations too high? It is unrealistic to expect a young baby to sleep for many hours without a feed, especially if you are breastfeeding, because breastmilk is digested more quickly than formula.

Your baby might settle more easily if he or she sleeps in the same room as an older sibling.

SHOULD YOU LEAVE A BABY TO CRY?

If you have a wakeful baby, then somebody may advise you to leave the baby to cry. But young babies are not old enough to assume that you are nearby. All they perceive is abandonment, so being left to cry may have a negative psychological effect. Even advocates of controlled crying say that sleep training shouldn't be tried with babies under the age of six months.

Gentle persuasion

If your baby tends to cry when put back down to sleep after a feed, he or she may want your company. If you want your baby to settle in the cot, try the following routine. You can also use this method to institute a regular bedtime. If the baby starts to cry at any point, revert to the previous action. You may find you have to run through the routine many, many times before your baby goes to sleep, but stay calm and persevere. Use the yoga exercise on the next page if you find yourself getting wound up, or let your partner take over. Don't feel you can't try again if you give up from time to time – if you repeat this routine regularly, your baby will eventually settle more easily.

1 When your baby cries, go in to the room, don't put on the light. Pick the baby up and soothe him or her with quiet shushing noises. As soon as the baby is calm, lay him or her gently in the cot again.

2 Keep one arm under the baby. Stroke the baby's tummy with the other hand still shushing. If you use a dummy (pacifier), give it to the baby. Slowly slide the arm out from under the baby, with the other hand on the tummy.

3 Continue shushing. Gradually decrease the stroking, but leave your hand resting there for a few moments longer. Slowly take away your hand, and gradually reduce the volume of your shushing.

4 Move slowly away from the cot, still quietly shushing, until you are out of the room. If your baby protests, go back and put your hand on his or her tummy. Repeat the process if you need to stop the baby getting upset.

Coping with broken nights

Sleepless nights are probably the hardest aspect of parenthood. Every parent feels tired at some point, and some find the first weeks and months disappear in a blur of exhaustion. Accept that you will get less sleep than before you had your baby – disturbed nights can be easier to deal with if you are relaxed about them. Some breastfeeding mothers say that they come to enjoy night feeds as a quiet time to share with their babies. Many parents feel pleased to see their baby, whatever the time. The following techniques can all help you to deal with being woken at night and minimize sleep deprivation.

- Have everything you may need in the night to hand: nappies, cotton wool (cotton balls), warm water in a flask, a spare sleepsuit for the baby; a bottle of water for you. You'll get back to sleep more quickly if you haven't had to go hunting around the house for these.
- Wear nightclothes so that you don't get cold if you get up and you don't have to scrabble around for a T-shirt when the baby is crying.

Being woken several times a night by your baby is hard. Keep fuss to the minimum by having everything you need to change the baby nearby.

Yoga relaxation exercise

This is a simple yoga pose that induces deep relaxation. You need at least ten minutes to relax fully. So it is best to do this exercise either when the baby has just gone down for a nap and is definitely asleep, or – better still – when there is somebody else in the house who can attend to the baby if he or she wakes.

Before you begin, make sure the room is warm and quiet – turn off any music, switch off the phone, close the curtains and ask anyone else in the house not to disturb you. Lie on a rug, yoga mat or large towel. You may like to cover yourself with a light blanket, and to put on some socks, to keep warm.

1 Sit on the floor, feet together and knees bent. Put your hands on either side of your buttocks. Slowly lie back, supporting your weight on your hands then elbows until you are lying flat, knees still bent. Lengthen the back of your neck as you put the back of your head on the floor. Stretch out your legs, feet apart.

2 If you feel discomfort in your lower back, place a cushion under your knees or leave them bent. Let your arms move comfortably out to your sides, palms upwards and fingers slightly curled. If your shoulders feel hunched, slide them down slightly. Close your eyes, relax and breathe for about ten minutes.

3 When you are ready to get up, bend your knees and roll over on to your left side. Come to a sitting position – taking your time – then get up slowly. Try to maintain slow steady breathing and a quiet frame of mind for a while. At the very least, don't instantly start to rush about.

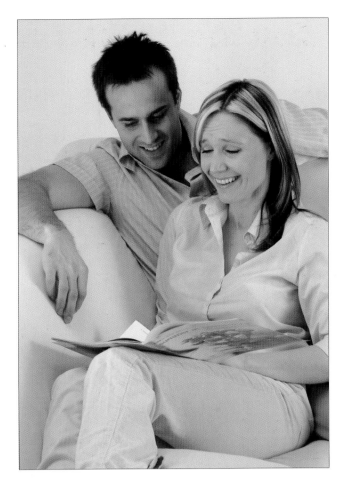

- Make yourself go to bed earlier than you might otherwise, even if you don't feel sleepy. If you find it hard to drop off, institute a nightly routine for yourself as well as for the baby. Have a warm bath, with a few drops of lavender or chamomile essential oil added to the water. Have a milky drink. Don't watch television in bed or read for long before sleep.
- During the day, grab a nap whenever the baby sleeps. Don't use the time to catch up on chores or phone calls if you are really tired; go to bed and rest. Even if you don't sleep, lying quietly will help replenish your energy.
- Eat well and healthily. Tiredness is harder to cope with if you are hungry.
- Practise deep breathing to calm the nervous system. Whenever you get a minute or two to yourself simply sit up straight, relax your shoulders and breathe.
- Consider taking time out to go to a yoga or pilates class. Check that the class is suitable for new mothers – ideally, go to a specialist class (you may be able to take the baby along or you may prefer to ask a friend, relative or your partner to babysit so that you can concentrate on your practice).
- Get out of the house at least once a day, even if you are feeling really tired. Fresh air and some kind of physical activity will do both you and the baby good and you may find the baby sleeps better at night if you provide plenty of stimulation during the day.

It is easy to get irritable when you are very tired, so take time to connect with your partner. Ask someone to take care of the baby to allow you to spend an hour or two alone together.

A drink of warm, cinnamon-spiced milk before you go to bed will help to relax you and encourage sleep.

DEVELOPING A NIGHTTIME STRATEGY

It's a good idea to have a strategy for dealing with broken nights. Discuss this with your partner in advance. It's much better to decide beforehand who is going to do what than to try and negotiate in the middle of the night when neither of you is likely to be feeling very reasonable.

Be realistic. Some partners may not be able or willing to do any nighttime parenting, especially if they have to get up early to go to work, and if you are breastfeeding, most of the night care will inevitably fall to you. Whatever strategy you have, there will be times when you need to be flexible. A father or helper can help at night in the following ways.

- If you are bottle-feeding, by giving a feed last thing at night. That way, you can go to bed earlier and get a few hours of unbroken sleep.
- By rocking or walking around with a baby who is ill or can't settle after being fed.
- By getting the baby up in the morning so that you can get an extra hour's sleep.
- By taking care of the baby in the early evening, to give you a break.

Some new fathers opt to spend nights sleeping in the spare room or on the sofa. This can help both of you in the short term – your partner gets a full night's sleep (which may make him better able to help you at other times) and you may sleep better if you have the bed to yourself. But obviously it is not something either of you will want to do for long.

Development and play

❝ Every baby is an individual: each one develops at his or her own pace and in a different way from any other. ❞

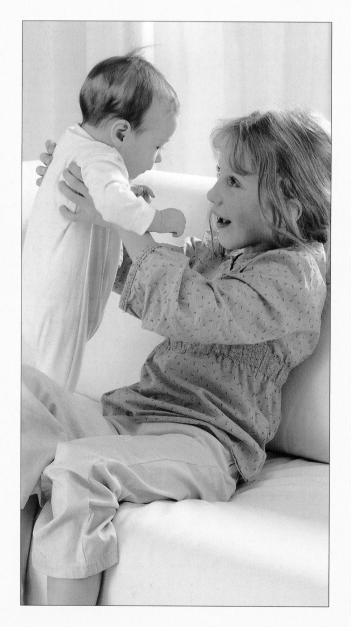

One of the real pleasures of parenthood is to watch your baby grow and develop. The tiny wriggling bundle you start with very soon becomes a fascinating child who sits up, laughs, babbles, and is curious about the world. Some changes happen suddenly – one day your baby is content to lie on a playmat, staring at a hanging toy; the next day he or she hits out at it. Other milestones, such as sitting up, take weeks of practice. And there are plateau periods, when your baby seems content simply to be. Doctors divide a baby's development into four key areas.

- Social development is about how your child interacts and responds to you and others, with smiles and little noises.
- Language development relates not only to how quickly and well a child learns to speak, but also to how much he or she understands what others say.
- Large motor development covers major physical actions such as sitting up, rolling over, crawling and walking.

The budding relationship between a baby and a sibling can be wonderful to watch. Babies often reward older children with the biggest smiles and belly laughs.

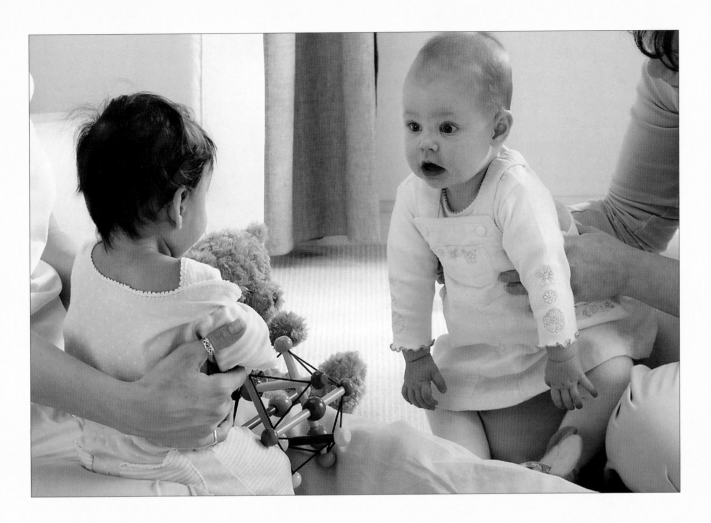

• Small motor development concerns more precise skills, including hand-to-eye coordination and the ability to hold and manipulate objects.

Health professionals will evaluate your baby's key achievements from time to time, to check that all is progressing normally. But if your child is late in developing certain skills, this doesn't necessarily mean there is something wrong. Every baby is an individual: each one develops at his or her own pace and in a different way. Some babies seem to learn new skills very easily, while others take longer to acquire them. Often a baby will be advanced in one area but late in others, and will forget about one skill for a while as he or she concentrates on learning something new.

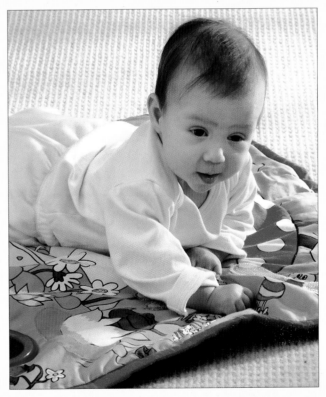

Top: Babies can be transfixed by other young children. At just a few months old, your baby may find another child much more fascinating than a new toy.

Your baby is preset to develop all the skills he or she needs. All you need to do is to provide him or her with a safe environment to explore.

Helping your baby to learn

B abies acquire new abilities when they are ready. As a parent, there isn't much that you can do to speed up this process. Pushing a child to learn a new skill before he or she is ready is at best pointless and at worst frustrating for you and potentially harmful for the child. However, you can make sure that your baby has a good environment for learning – one that is loving, stimulating and encouraging.

Babies are born with a drive to explore the world around them. The way they learn best is through human interaction, so lots of love and attention is what a baby needs most. Talk directly to your baby, sing to him or her, explain what is going on. Describe what you are doing as you, say, change a nappy, and point out interesting things when you are out together. Your baby won't understand the words you are using, of course, but will pick up on your interest and respond to it.

Until your baby can walk around and explore, you have to bring the world to the baby. Offer interesting things to look at and let the baby touch them. If you are looking at a plant in the garden, say, hold the baby close enough to reach out and grab it. Gently brush different materials – silk, cotton wool, corduroy – across the baby's skin to help him or her learn about texture.

Give your baby interesting things to smell, such as a citrus fruit or a lavender bag. Let the baby hold your watch or a sturdy necklace when sitting on your lap. From a few months old, your baby will start to put everything in his or her mouth: this is not an attempt to eat things, but an infant's primary mode of investigating physical objects.

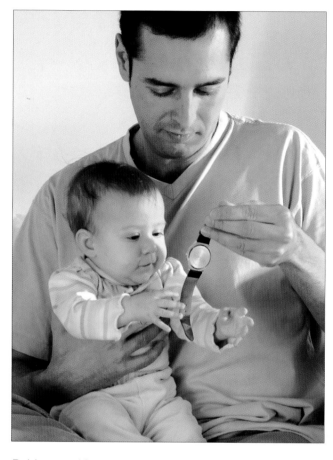

Babies need human company in order to develop well. A baby who spends hours each day in a cot or bouncy chair, without anything interesting to look at, will become bored and understimulated.

Sometimes a baby doesn't need a toy or other entertainment, he or she will be quite happy just watching you and following your movements.

While babies love to play with their parents, siblings and other close people, they don't need to be actively entertained all the time.

DEVELOPMENTAL MILESTONES

Keep a relaxed attitude to your baby's development. Most parents look at developmental charts at some time or other, and it is very easy to worry if your baby hasn't achieved a so-called "milestone" at the usual time. If your baby seems to be very late, or has missed several milestones, then discuss this with a health professional. But don't get too hung up on whether your child is "advanced" or "behind". The ages given for developmental milestones are simply statistical averages of certain easily observable behaviours. They are not an exam your baby has to pass. Reaching the stages early does not mean your child is phenomenally clever, and reaching them late does not imply anything about future academic achievement. Albert Einstein, one of the most incisive and original minds of the 20th century, was a "slow" child who did not start to talk until he was three.

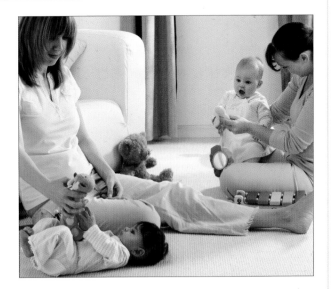

Mixing with other parents and babies gives you a good idea of how babies develop at different rates.

Lots of cuddles help babies to feel secure, and give a sense of a "base" from which to explore their surroundings. But that doesn't mean they have to be held all the time. In fact, it is good to let your baby see things from different positions. Put the Moses basket or pram in a variety of places where there are interesting things to look at. Lay the baby on his or her front sometimes, so that he or she gets a new viewpoint and can practise different movements such as lifting the head.

FOLLOW THE BABY

Tailor playtime to your baby's temperament, likes and dislikes. Some babies are very active from a young age and enjoy being tickled, say, or bounced up and down. Others are more nervous and prefer gentler play. It is important to be sensitive to your baby and not to persist with games that make him or her unhappy or scared. Similarly, don't let anyone else play with your baby in this way – it is quite common for men, in particular, to play rough games with baby boys in the mistaken belief that this will toughen them up. If your baby doesn't seem to be enjoying a game, put a stop to it.

Always follow your baby's lead. If he or she is enjoying a particular toy, don't try to introduce another one. Let the baby explore this one fully, show him or her what it does, and join in the game.

Try to pitch activities at your baby's level, or just above it. This makes playtime stimulating but fun. If your baby is

Introduce your baby to different textures by stroking fabric over his or her tummy or palm. Try something soft such as a square of velvet or a furry soft toy, and see how the baby reacts.

taking an interest in a particular toy, say, you could play peek-a-boo with it. The baby will appreciate the surprise and will soon learn that things are still there even when they can't be seen – a key human attribute. If the baby likes to hold a particular rattle, next time try offering one that is a different shape, size or colour to explore.

Be aware of your baby's moods. If he or she is hungry it is time for a feed, not playtime. And even when happily enjoying a toy, a baby won't want to play with it for more than a few minutes. Starting to cry, turning away or getting a glazed look are signs that the baby has had enough: follow these cues.

Above all, mark your baby's tiny successes with enthusiasm. Babies, like the rest of us, like to be encouraged. Use exaggerated facial expressions and a joyous tone of voice. Your smiles, claps and exclamations of "Clever baby!" will delight your child and make him or her want to try new things.

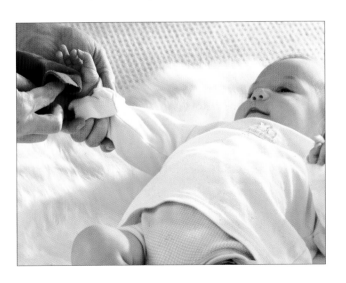

Seeing and hearing

People used to think that newborns were deaf and blind, but we now know that babies can see and hear from birth. Their vision is poor at first, but they can see almost as well as adults by the time they are eight months old. Hearing is the most developed sense in a newborn and is almost perfect by the time the baby is a month old.

SIGHT

The vision of newborn babies is limited and blurred, but they can focus on things that are 20–30cm/8–12in away. Faces are what interest babies most at this stage, but they will also be transfixed by simple patterns that have good contrast – try showing your baby simple black and white geometrical designs.

By two months, babies are able to track a moving object with both eyes. They are just starting to be able to distinguish colours at this point – they may show an interest in bright primary colours as well as more complicated patterns. This can be a good time to begin to show a baby colourful board books.

Babies start to get a sense of perspective by about four months, and this helps them with their new-found grasping skills. They are now able to focus on small

New babies are unaware of their hands, but suddenly they discover these fascinating things belong to them.

Check it out

Your baby's vision and hearing will be checked at routine developmental reviews, but it is important to see a doctor if you think your baby is not responding to sound or that there may be a problem with his or her sight. Many problems are easier to correct if they are picked up early on. You can check your child's hearing in the following ways, but don't panic if your baby doesn't respond: he or she may just be absorbed in something else, or be tired and distracted. Don't keep going; just give up and try again another time.

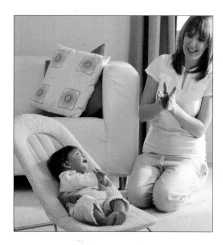

0–3 months: Clap your hands behind a baby's head (not by an ear). If the baby reacts, hearing is normal.

4–6 months: Call your baby's name to see if he or she turns to you. Babies of this age should also turn towards the source of an unusual sound – try tapping on a glass with a fork or making a squeaking noise.

Babies are born with perfect pitch and enjoy listening to all manner of soothing sounds – such as a ticking clock or a set of wind chimes.

Babies are fascinated by shiny objects that catch the light. Try holding up a length of foil and watching your baby react.

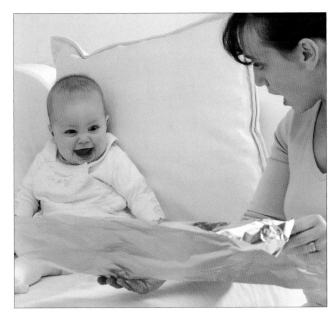

objects as well as large ones. Over the next month or so, they begin to spot small items from farther away, and get better at tracking moving objects. They also find it easier to distinguish between different colours.

HEARING

The sense of hearing develops in the womb, and there is evidence to suggest that babies can hear sounds outside the womb as early as 25 weeks. One study found that newborns could recognize the theme tune of the Australian soap opera *Neighbours* if their mothers had watched it regularly while pregnant.

From birth, babies are interested in human voices: they show a preference for their native language and they prefer their mother's voice to anyone else's. They also respond more keenly to high-pitched tones than low ones – most people sense this and automatically assume a higher pitch when they talk to babies. But even though your baby is listening intently to you, he or she may not turn towards you when you speak until the age of about three months. Babies also show an innate appreciation of music; they enjoy soothing music from birth, and they seem to prefer songs to purely instrumental music.

FIVE GOOD TOYS FOR YOUNG BABIES

Newborns babies don't need toys, but by three or four weeks old your baby will be able to appreciate some of the following.

Mobile. A mobile makes a wonderful amusement. Hang it within easy focusing distance – ideally, about 25cm/10in away – and to the baby's right or left (babies usually lie with their head pointing to one side rather than upwards). Babies can't distinguish between colours until they are three months old, so choose one that has sharp contrasts – either black and white or bold colours.

Mirror. Babies are fascinated by their own reflection – although they don't understand that they are looking at themselves until they are well over a year old. Choose soft toys or books that have a special unbreakable mirror attached.

Black-and-white patterns. A new baby will be fascinated by geometric black-and-white patterns, and you should be able to find cloth books or soft toys that use these designs. Alternatively, draw some simple designs on paper and stick these to the wall next to the Moses basket.

Rattle. Babies are interested in noises so they like playing with rattles. Moving a rattle around helps to make the connection between cause and effect, as the baby learns that shaking the rattle makes a noise.

Baby gym. A baby gym can give your child months of pleasure. When lying on his or her front there are different textures, colours and sometimes sounds to enjoy. Lying on his or her back, the baby has space to kick around and toys to look at, swipe and grasp. Hang the toys in different places so that there are different ones to reach for.

How movement develops

Newborns aren't able to control their movements, and any seemingly purposeful movements they make – such as sucking or grasping – are due to survival reflexes. However, both before and after birth babies will kick, fling out their arms and twist their bodies. These simple random movements strengthen the muscles and stimulate the nervous system. Gradually, your baby learns how to lift and move different parts of his or her body.

The development of motor control follows a set pattern in all babies: it moves from the top downwards and from the centre outwards. So, babies will learn to hold up their head long before they can move their legs. And they will use their arms to hit out at an object before they can close their hand in order to hold it.

HEAD CONTROL

In very young babies, the neck muscles are too weak to hold up the heavy head, so you need to support it whenever you hold your baby. By six weeks, there is some degree of head control: when held, babies start to lift their head up for a few seconds at a time, and may move it from side to side. They can keep their head steady when sitting in an infant carrier or a bouncy chair.

When they lie on their tummy, three-month-old babies will lift their head off the floor and turn it so that they can look around – a few babies are strong enough to do this when they are just a few weeks old. They won't do it for long at first, but as their strength grows, they'll start lifting up on their hands so that their shoulders come up too. This is an important precursor to crawling.

By four months, your baby will be able to keep his or her head up as you carry him or her around (though you may still need to support the head if you are performing an awkward manoeuvre, such as getting the baby into a

Head control develops very slowly, so you need to support your baby's head for several months. But he or she will try to lift the head from an early age.

car seat). And by six months most babies have developed neck muscles strong enough to keep themselves upright if their lower bodies are supported. Soon they will be able to sit up by themselves; some already can at this age.

ROCKING AND ROLLING

The first independent movement babies make is rolling (usually from their front on to their back). Instead of lying wherever you have placed your baby, he or she discovers how to get a toy that is just out of reach or change his or her viewpoint. It's hugely exciting for both of you, and once your baby has mastered the skill, he or she will roll at every opportunity. Babies sometimes roll from front to back as early as two months, but rolling from back to front takes greater control of the head and arms. It usually happens between five and seven months.

Because rolling sometimes happens without warning, it is essential that you never leave a baby unattended on a high surface (such as a bed or changing table). Don't turn away for a second.

TRYING TO SIT

Babies start trying to sit up from three or four months, once they have some head control. If you lay babies of this age on their back, they may lift up their head so that

The first step towards rolling over is when a baby starts to crane the head while lying on the back. It takes many practice goes before he or she manages to flip over.

Encouraging rolling

Like all physical skills, rolling happens when your baby is ready. But you can encourage back to front rolling with a toy that they reach for. Make sure he or she is lying on a flat surface – a crumpled blanket will impede movement.

1 Lie your baby on his or her back. Attract your baby's attention by holidng a favourite toy above him or her, just out of reach.

2 Hold the toy away to one side to encourage the baby to stretch towards it, and begin to rock on to his or her side.

3 Gently hold the baby on his or her side for a few moments. Then slowly turn the baby on to his or her front, making sure he or she is happy.

Encouraging Sitting

Babies start trying to sit up from an early age. But they have to develop neck muscles strong enough to support the head. When this happens, your baby will enjoy being pulled to a sitting position.

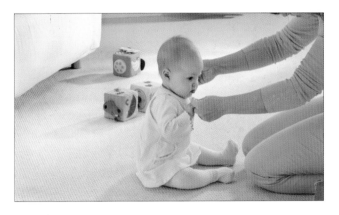

1 Wait until your baby is lying on his or her back. Offer the baby your hands and see if he or she tries to rise up. If so, you can gently help him or her come to a sitting position. Make sure that the neck stays in line with the body.

2 From a sitting position, you can slowly lower your baby back onto their back. Again, make sure that the neck is in line with the body. A few well-judged sound-effects – "dooooown", "uuuuuuup" – will make it more fun.

they can look around. If you give them your hands, they'll try to pull themselves up to a sitting position.

Babies enjoy being propped up so that they can see what is going on around them. A bouncy chair is ideal for this, especially one that can be adjusted from an almost reclining position to a more upright one as the baby's head control improves. When the neck and back muscles have strengthened to the extent that your baby is nearly sitting up (usually at about five or six months), you can use an L-shaped breastfeeding cushion or ordinary pillows to support him or her. Make sure that there are cushions all around so that the baby isn't hurt if he or she falls forward or sideways.

As soon as they master some head control, babies love to sit up and watch what is going on around them. Prop your baby up on some cushions for brief periods, but as he or she will inevitably slip gradually downwards, you'll have to be there to make sure he or she stays upright and doesn't topple over.

Fun with movement

All babies really need for the development of large motor control is a safe space to move about in. If they are always in a bouncy chair, sling or pushchair, they won't be able to learn how their body moves. So, give your baby plenty of time on the floor where he or she can enjoy a good wriggle around.

You can help your baby to practise his or her new-found muscle control by playing physical games. Always

From about six weeks, put your baby on his or her tummy often to practise lifting his or her head, which will strengthen the neck muscles. A few minutes a day is all that is needed. Sit on the floor close by and chat to encourage your baby to look up at you.

Babies love using their bodies. 'Bicycling' is a great way to help them experience a different movement.

be gentle and do what your baby seems to enjoy. When the baby is lying on his or her back, try bicycling: move the legs alternately towards the body, bending them into the chest and then stretching them out towards you. Lift the baby up into the air and move him or her around before bringing him or her back to the safety of your lap.

Give your baby lots of tummy time so that he or she can practise lifting up the head and upper body. Some babies don't like going on their tummies, but there are lots of ways you can make this fun. Get down there too,

Ball play

This little game of catch will keep your baby amused during his or her tummy time. It is also good exercise for the neck, arm and leg muscles, making it a good preparation for crawling. Stop as soon as your baby seems uncomfortable.

1 When your baby lifts his or her head, roll a ball about 60cm/2 ft in front of him or her. At first the baby will be content just to watch it move.

2 As he or she gets stronger, the baby will reach out to grab the ball as it rolls. Give lots of praise whenever this happens.

3 Always end the game by giving your baby the ball to play with. He or she is more likely to stay interested in a game than ends in success.

Baby yoga: wind-relieving posture

This aptly named yoga pose works on the digestive system and helps a baby to release any trapped wind. If your baby is windy or colicky, it is a good one to include in a massage routine, or you can just do it by itself.

1 Place your baby on a blanket on the floor. Holding the baby's knees, open his or her legs out so that the knees are wider than the hips.

2 Slowly bring the knees to touch the body. Make the movement smooth and relaxed. Release the pressure, and then repeat twice more.

3 Keeping the baby's knees bent, bring the legs over to the left. Hold for a moment, pressing the knees gently into the side of the abdomen.

4 Release the pressure and slowly return the legs to the centre. Move them to the right and hold against the side of the abdomen. Repeat twice.

so that your baby doesn't feel scared: make eye contact, talk or sing, and make silly expressions to keep him or her amused. Use a playmat that has different textures and colours to explore. Place a mirror in front of the baby so that pushing up is rewarded by his or her own face.

Hold your baby under the arms so that he or she can "stand" on your lap; the baby will push down to straighten his or her legs and may enjoy bouncing up and down. Once he or she has good head control (at about five or six months) the baby will probably appreciate being in a baby bouncer for short periods. Some babies who can raise themselves up on their arms when lying on their front enjoy the "wheelbarrow" position: try lifting your baby's legs, then lowering them back down and repeating. Show the baby you are excited by these achievements by exclaiming, smiling and making plenty of eye contact.

BABY YOGA

Yoga helps babies to learn about and enjoy their bodies. If you are interested in baby yoga it is worth going to classes, but you can also do some simple movements at home. Babies are naturally flexible, so the postures are more like massage techniques than exercise, and you can easily incorporate them into a baby massage routine. But it is very important to be gentle; never force a movement or persist with the poses if your baby seems unhappy.

Baby yoga; butterfly pose

This is an adaptation of another favourite yoga pose, which works on the hips and pelvis.

Babies have very flexible hip joints so they love this movement. Hold both your baby's ankles with your hands. Move the feet together so that the soles are touching. Gently push the feet into the abdomen, hold for a moment and then release. Then try pushing the legs slowly in and out in a rhythmic way.

CLASSES FOR BABIES

Baby classes of some kind are available in most areas. You could easily sign your baby up to a curriculum that involves baby yoga, baby gymnastics and baby swimming, as well as baby signing and baby music. All these can be fun. But be selective: cramming lots of classes into your baby's schedule may make him or her tired and cranky.

If you do choose to go to a class, pick one that feels relaxed and fun. Avoid any that make excessive promises about baby development, or that seem to foster a competitive spirit. Above all, don't feel that you are depriving your baby if you don't join any classes. Your baby can learn just as much at home, on simple outings and in parent-and-baby groups.

Handling and chewing

Newborn babies are born with the grasping reflex but it takes months before they can reach for an object and pick it up. During the first weeks of life, babies' hands are curled into fists. They may hold a small toy if they are given it, but won't really explore it for some weeks to come. At about eight weeks, your baby may start to hit out at objects, such as the items hanging on a play gym, or toys attached to the bouncy chair or pram. It is a good idea to make sure they are within arm's length, so that the baby doesn't become frustrated. At this stage, babies play with their own hands from time to time, but they don't yet realize that they actually belong to them – they won't look at their hands unless they happen to be in their line of vision.

From about eight weeks, babies start to open their hands. If given a small toy to play with, they will instinctively grasp it and may finger it for a little while. A noisy toy, such as a rattle, is ideal because the sound it makes will draw a baby's attention to his or her hands. By three months, babies' hands are their favourite playthings. They examine them intently, put them in their mouth, bring them together and apart again. They also enjoy batting toys within reach, and occasionally manage to grab hold of one.

All this activity helps to develop hand-to-eye coordination. By three or four months, babies can pick up large objects they see and will deliberately grasp a toy

A small wooden toy with moving parts like this one is perfect for fingering, and will keep your baby entertained for several minutes at a time.

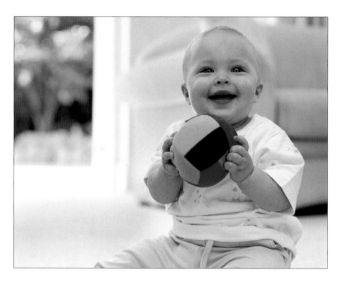

A soft ball can be grabbed easily and provides an interesting texture to explore. If it has a bell inside, then the amusement factor is even greater.

that is held out to them. Make sure that you give your baby the time he or she needs to reach out, though, as it can take a baby a little while to respond. Try using a squeaky toy to add to the fun.

Once babies can hold objects, they will put them in their mouth. The mouth has more nerve endings than the fingertips, so it is the best tool for exploration. This means that everything within reach of your baby should be safe for sucking. Don't give a baby anything that could be toxic or allow him or her to handle anything small enough to choke on (such as a string of beads).

By six months, babies can pass a toy from one hand to the other and reach for an object without looking at their hands as they do so. And they can work out whether a toy is within reach or not – they won't try to grab it if it is too far away.

GOOD TOYS FOR GRASPING
When your baby is at the swiping stage, hang an interesting mobile so that the items are within batting distance. A play gym is excellent for this, especially if you can move the toys around to keep up the baby's interest. Your baby can play with other things besides toys, of course. Household objects that have no sharp edges – such as a whisk, a set of measuring spoons or some plastic pots – are ideal for your tiny explorer. Once your baby can take hold of things, provide a range of toys to explore, including different sizes, textures, sounds and shapes, such as the following.

- Toys that have small protrusions for easy grabbing.
- Toys with two handles for passing from hand to hand.
- Toys that a baby can safely put in his or her mouth – this is good for teething.
- Toys that are brightly coloured with sharp contrasts.
- Toys that are interesting to feel – squishy fabric blocks, smooth plastic objects, soft toys, toys that have contrasting textures.
- Toys that make any kind of a noise, such as rattles and squeaky toys.

GRASPING GAME

A good game you can play to encourage grasping is to attach a brightly coloured soft toy to a piece of string or ribbon. Prop your baby up in a sitting position and then dangle it in front of him of her. When the baby reaches for it, say "Well done," with lots of smiles. Always end the game by giving the toy to the baby to play with, but detach the string or ribbon first.

TOYS AND SAFETY

Make sure that anything your baby plays with is safe. In particular make sure you follow these guidelines:
- A toy should not be small enough to fit completely into the baby's mouth.
- There should no detachable parts that are small enough to choke on.
- It should be lightweight, so that it will not hurt if your baby drops it on to his or her face when lying down.
- It should be made of non-toxic materials.
- A soft toy should be machine- or surface-washable. Check that the seams are securely sewn and make sure there are no trimmings, such as eyes, noses, buttons or ribbons that can be pulled or bitten off.
- All toys should meet the recognized safety standards.
- Don't give a toy that is intended for an older child to

From two or three months, babies can hold objects and will lift them up to their mouths to suck. Small items of kitchen equipment hold as much fascination as any toy – try giving your baby a set of plastic measuring spoons, or a wooden spoon to explore.

your baby. Toys are labelled with recommended ages for safety reasons.
- Don't give a balloon to a baby. It may burst, which will be frightening, and if a small part of the balloon is swallowed it may cause choking.
- Don't attach a toy to a cot or pram with string or ribbon.
- Remove mobiles and other hanging objects once a baby begins to push up on hands or knees.

Once your baby can sit, he or she will enjoy knocking down a tower of bricks that you have built.

Encourage your baby to grasp by holding out a toy. If he or she reaches for it, give it to them.

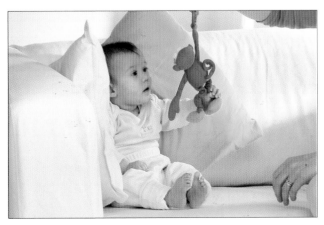

Sociability and language

Babies are social beings. Right from the start they need company, and are happiest when they are getting plenty of cuddles. Young babies don't have a sense of being a separate person – they don't know their hands are their own, for example, and they can't tell where their mother's body ends and theirs begins. They just instinctively know that it is good to be around people.

Young babies like to look at faces more than anything else, but they can't at first tell the difference between a real face and a picture, and they cannot recognize expression: a scary face is just as interesting and enjoyable to a tiny baby as a smiling one.

By about three months babies can recognize individuals, and will smile more readily at those they know well – their mother, father, siblings and so on. Over the next weeks and months, they become increasingly attached to their main carer. This is usually the mother, but if both parents share the care – or if a grandparent or childminder is very involved in the child's life – then the baby will naturally develop strong attachments to those people too.

But babies are also interested in new people. It's a good idea to give your baby plenty of opportunities to meet people, and to let him or her engage with relatives, friends and people that you come into contact with when you are out. This helps to foster the notion that the world is a friendly place – which is good for socialization skills.

First smiles are a response to a familiar voice. It's not until about eight or nine weeks that a baby will smile when you smile. When he or she realizes that smiling gets attention and cuddles, the baby does it a lot more.

Your baby will learn to speak by listening to your voice and copying you. It will help if you make eye contact, and give him or her a chance to respond.

BABY TALK

At first your baby communicates only through crying, but after the first weeks, he or she will start to coo and gurgle. The first sounds – "aah", "eeeh" and other vowel sounds – will be random at first. But soon you will notice that the baby coos at you or at a particular object that has captured his or her attention.

Your baby will also start making easily articulated consonant sounds – "ma", "da" and "ba". Some babies do this as early as three months, some not until six months. Whatever age they start, they enjoy practising their new sounds. They also love it if you make the same sounds to them – try it and see how your baby reacts. Gradually babies start babbling: practising strings of consonant sounds such as "babababa", "dadadada", "mamama", over and over. Six months is an average age to do this – but many babies will do it considerably later.

By now, you'll be waiting for your baby to say "Mama" or "Dada". Lots of babies can do this at about eight months, and "Dada" usually comes first. But they won't use these words to mean their parents for another few months to come.

As well as practising sounds, babies start to laugh at about three and a half months. They also learn to screech to attract your attention. Don't worry that you are teaching bad habits when you respond to a deliberate scream – your baby will adopt different ways of calling you as soon as he or she is able.

GOOD WAYS TO TALK TO YOUR BABY

- Read to your baby from a young age. Look at a brightly coloured picture book together and make up your own words. Read the same story again and again. Give your baby cloth and tough board books that can safely be chewed.

- Play games – count your baby's toes and play "This little piggy" on them, play "Round and round the garden" on his or her palm and "Incy-wincy spider" on the baby's tummy.
- Recite nursery rhymes. If you have forgotten the words, buy or borrow a children's book.
- Sing to your baby often. Play lots of music too – classical music helps to stimulate areas of the brain that deal with literacy and numeracy.

- Have "conversations". Even very young babies move their mouths, as if trying to speak. Respond to this with "How interesting", "That's a good story" and so on.
- When your baby starts to makes sounds, copy them – you'll get a smile when you do. Remember to pause so that the baby can "answer" you.
- Point out things of interest when you are out and

about. Name common objects – "cow", "car", "flower" – as the more often your baby hears words in context the more quickly he or she will learn them. Talk about whatever you are doing – changing or bathing your baby, say.

A baby will observe your face closely, so make exaggerated expressions when you talk to him or her. Try opening your mouth and sticking out your tongue – even a very new baby may copy you.

repetition are helpful: they serve to reiterate the main sounds of the words, giving babies a second chance to hear them and commit them to memory. Diminutive endings – "teethies", "doggies" – are another universal element of baby talk: this way of speaking is also helpful, as "framing" the consonant sound between vowels makes it easier to hear and learn. So don't feel embarrassed about lapsing into baby talk when you chat to your child – you are just doing what comes naturally.

BILINGUAL BABIES

Learning to speak is a fantastic intellectual achievement – one that all babies accomplish by the age of three. Strange as it may seem, it is no harder for a baby to learn two languages than one. So, if you and your partner speak different languages, each of you should stick to your own. Your baby will assume that there is a mummy language and a daddy language and will rise magnificently to the challenge of acquiring both.

HOW TO TALK TO YOUR CHILD

Some people find it very easy to chat to their babies; others think it is pointless talking to a baby who cannot understand them. But talking gives babies emotional stability, and it helps with language development and learning. Children learn their native language because they hear other people using it, so you have to give them the "raw data" to work with.

Most people naturally adopt a pitch higher than normal when talking to babies, as they are more responsive to this. "Baby talk" also includes lots of rhymes – such as "milky-wilky" and "itty-bitty" – and repetitive elements – "night-night", "bye-bye". Both rhyme and simple

It's great if your baby is happy to go to other people for a cuddle, but he or she will always want to come back to you. You may also notice that your baby grabs at your face and pokes his or her fingers in your mouth with great gusto, but is a lot more restrained when held by someone less familiar.

section two

your older baby

six months to one year

The experience of caring for a small baby is a mixture of anxiety and joy. But gradually, as you become seasoned parents, the joy starts to predominate and everything seems much easier to accomplish. You will be astonished by the rate at which your baby changes during his or her second six months. You can almost literally see him or her grow and develop before your eyes, and little by little a distinctive and individual personality begins to emerge.

General care and feeding

66 It is immensely satisfying to know that you are training your baby's palate, laying the foundations for a lifetime of healthy eating. 99

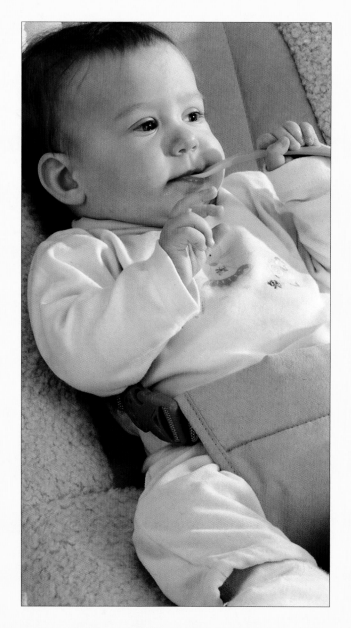

By now you will be better accustomed to caring for your baby and will be able to meet his or her basic needs with a more practised ease: long gone are the days when you struggled to get that sleepsuit over tiny arms and legs.

But babies grow fast and parenthood brings with it an ever-changing set of challenges. Around the six-month mark, your baby will start to cut his or her first teeth. Some babies do this without seeming to notice it; others feel a lot of pain and require lots of gentle aid to help them through the teething process.

The advent of teeth is a sign that your baby is getting ready for real food. Don't be surprised if you find it hard to give up the deep connection that comes with breastfeeding: this is a normal feeling. It is one of the many acts of letting go that are integral to parenthood. If you are committed to providing your baby with natural food, you will find that the changeover to solids involves a great deal of work at first: there are all those fruits and vegetables to cook, purée and pour into ice-cube trays for freezing. But it

Your baby may find a first experience of solid food strange, but he or she will soon get the taste for it and may grab the spoon out of your hand.

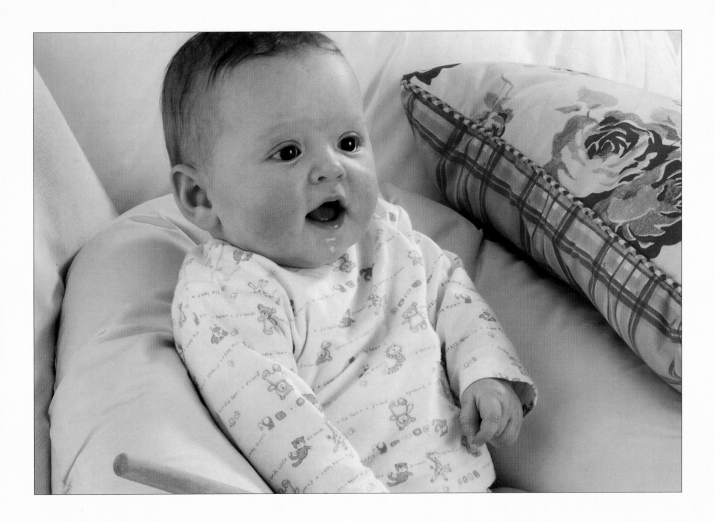

is also immensely satisfying to know that you are helping to train your baby's palate, laying the foundations for a lifetime of healthy eating. And, like all aspects of childcare, feeding your baby gets much easier with practice.

Many women return to work in their baby's first year, for perfectly good reasons, but if you find that you cannot bear to leave your baby after all, you are not alone. It's worth considering whether you can extend the time you spend together by negotiating more flexible working hours, for example. But if you do need to go back to work, for whatever reason, you will naturally want to choose your childcare carefully. Leaving your baby is much easier once you are confident that he or she is being looked after lovingly by someone you trust.

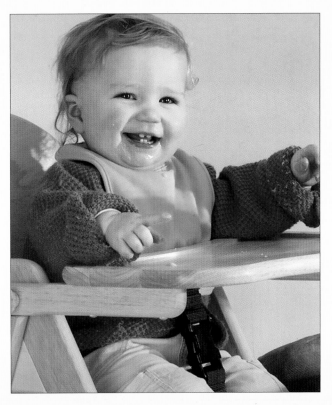

Top: Your baby will be much more aware of, and entertained by, his or her surroundings, and will watch your face and activities with absorbed interest.

Weaning is fun. There is huge pleasure to be had in introducing a baby to new flavours and seeing his or her growing enjoyment of good food.

Teething and tooth care

Spotting that tiny white line on your baby's gum is an exciting event – the first tooth is on its way. This can happen at any time in the first year, but teeth usually start coming through when a baby is around six months old.

WHEN THE TEETH COME THROUGH

Baby teeth tend to come through in pairs in a set sequence. But your baby's teeth may emerge in a slightly different order to the one described here, and they may appear earlier or later than the average ages given. They will look crooked when they are coming through, but will soon straighten out. Eventually your baby will have 20 milk teeth (compared to an adult's 32 permanent teeth).

TEETHING PAIN

The first teeth are sharp, thin incisors, so they usually cut through the gum quite easily. But if your baby is cutting more than one tooth at once, or if one of the large flat molars is emerging, this can cause a lot of discomfort.

To help your baby cope with the teething process, try rubbing the gums with a clean finger or a finger-toothbrush. You may be able to feel a bump on the gum before a tooth comes through. Something cool to bite on can help: a smooth hard toy or a clean facecloth dipped in cold water both work well, or you can use a teething ring that's been cooled in the fridge (not the freezer). Some people find that a stick of peeled carrot, a breadstick or a sugar-free teething biscuit helps; stay close by in case your baby manages to bite off a bit. You

A few babies are actually born with teeth, while others don't develop any until after they are a year old.

can also breastfeed for comfort. Teething babies often want to nurse more frequently and need lots of fluid.

Many babies find homeopathic teething granules (Chamomilla) very soothing. But if natural methods don't seem to work, try rubbing teething gel on the gum. This numbs the area and can help a baby get off to sleep, but it is suitable only for babies over the age of about four months. You can also give your baby infant paracetamol (acetaminophen) to help with pain and reduce any fever.

This is a general guide to when you can expect which of your baby's teeth to appear.

Get your baby a toothbrush as soon as the first tooth comes through.

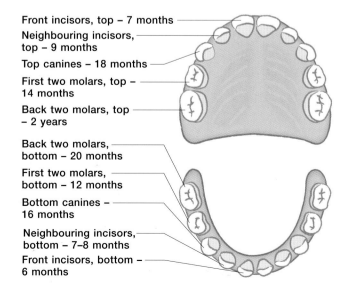

Front incisors, top – 7 months

Neighbouring incisors, top – 9 months

Top canines – 18 months

First two molars, top – 14 months

Back two molars, top – 2 years

Back two molars, bottom – 20 months

First two molars, bottom – 12 months

Bottom canines – 16 months

Neighbouring incisors, bottom – 7–8 months

Front incisors, bottom – 6 months

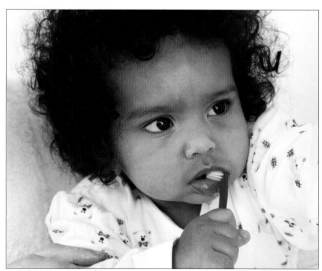

PROTECTING YOUR BABY'S TEETH

- Don't give your baby any sugary foods.
- Limit dried fruit to an occasional treat.
- Limit drinks to water and milk only.
- Always use sugar-free medicines.
- Take your baby with you when you go to the dentist for your own check-ups, so that the surgery becomes familiar. Always talk about going to the dentist in a positive and enthusiastic way.

TOOTH CARE

Start cleaning your baby's teeth as soon as the first ones come through. You'll find this easier if you lay the baby on your lap so that you are looking down at his or her mouth. If your baby doesn't like you using a baby toothbrush, try using a piece of damp gauze wrapped around your finger. Put a tiny smear of toothpaste on the gauze and clean the teeth very gently using circular movements, twice a day.

Don't worry if your baby won't let you brush his or her teeth at all; just give the brush to the baby to chew on. So long as you are using a fluoride toothpaste, this will help to strengthen the teeth and protect them from decay. It is important not to let tooth cleaning become stressful. At this stage it should be enjoyable and fun; but once several teeth are through they will need to be cleaned.

THE RIGHT TOOTHPASTE

Most dentists recommend that you use a specially formulated children's fluoride toothpaste for your baby. Adult toothpaste contains higher levels of fluoride, so it is not suitable: too much fluoride can cause discoloration of

Babies are fascinated by toothbrushing. Try giving your baby his or her own brush at the same time as you use yours, to copy you. Let your baby have a go at "brushing" your teeth while you are cleaning his or hers.

CHECKLIST: IS YOUR BABY TEETHING?

Be careful not to confuse real illness with signs of teething. If your baby seems to be in real pain, has a high temperature, a rash, diarrhoea or other symptoms, see a doctor. The following are the classic signs of teething.

Dribbling: More saliva is produced, so your baby is likely to dribble a lot more than usual. Many babies get a runny nose as well.

Distress and irritability. Pain will make your baby fractious and possibly more clingy than usual.

Biting and gnawing. Pressure on the gum relieves the pain so your baby may want to chew on everything (including you). The baby may bite his or her bottom lip before the first teeth come through.

Swelling on the gum. The gum may look red, bumpy or sore.

Flushed cheek. One or both cheeks may be red.

Fever. A slightly raised temperature is common with teething, especially at night.

Nappy rash. Many babies produce runny stools and are prone to nappy rash when teething.

Wakefulness. The baby may wake up more than usual at night.

the teeth. Fluoride is a mineral found in water. Additional fluoride is added to the water supply of some British regions and almost all US states to improve dental health. If there are only low levels of fluoride in your water, you may consider giving your baby a fluoride supplement, but you must take advice on this from a dentist: you could damage your child's teeth if you give too much fluoride.

Bikkie pegs are natural, rock hard, teething chews that some babies enjoy gnawing on.

Homeopathic teething granules don't ease pain, but have a soothing effect on any fretfulness.

Bathing and dressing an older baby

Bathtime is a lot more fun once your baby is old enough to enjoy toys, games and lots of splashing in the big bath. Most older babies love having a bath, and a soak in warm water can be an excellent way of calming them down before bedtime. But having a bath straight after a meal can make a baby sick so leave a gap.

Make sure the bathroom is very warm and have a towel ready so that you can wrap your baby up as soon as you lift him or her out of the water. Until your baby is a confident sitter, you will have to lean over to support him or her throughout bathtime. This is hard on your back: make sure you are facing the bath squarely so that you are not twisting it.

BATHTIME GAMES

The best way to get your baby enjoying water is by playing in the bathtub.

- Lay your baby down on his or her back in the water, supporting the head and bottom, and swoosh him or her up and down the bath. Then turn the baby over and do the same, this time with your hands under the chin and tummy.
- Scoop water up in a beaker and pour it gently over the baby's tummy. Hold the beaker high and pour water into the bath in front of the baby so that it makes a glistening stream. He or she will reach out and touch it.

If your baby stops wanting to go in the bath, try getting in too. Take extra care when you are getting in and out, or have someone else there to lift the baby out for you.

BABY BATH OIL
To give your baby a beautifully aromatic and calming bath before bedtime, add a few drops of oil scented with mandarin orange to the water. Combine ten drops of mandarin essential oil with 100ml/3½fl oz sunflower oil, and store in a dark glass bottle out of direct sunlight. This oil will keep for 12 months.

- Gently trickle water on the baby's face using a facecloth or a scoop toy. This should help your baby to cope with any splashing in the pool if you go swimming together.
- Get some bath toys to play with. A natural sponge is great fun, and your baby will enjoy filling and emptying stacking cups or plastic bowls and beakers.
- If you have an older child, let them take a bath together – your baby will love playing in the water with a big brother or sister.

WASHING YOUR BABY

It is best to avoid baby bath products that contain chemicals, since these strip the natural oils from your baby's skin. You don't usually need to "wash" your baby at this age anyway: you can do without shampoo, soap and bubble bath. If your baby has some grubby patches, you can use an oatmeal "sponge": simply put a handful of oats in a muslin square, and twist to make a pouch. Water dries out the skin, so add a little oil to the bath. And of course, you don't have to bath your baby every day; a daily sponge bath of face, neck, underarms, hands, nappy area and feet is enough to keep a baby clean.

Babies love water games, and a natural sponge and a few simple toys add to the fun of bathtime.

Left: Your baby will enjoy your cry of "Where's baby?" as his or her face disappears inside a top, and your start of surprise when a face is revealed. Play peek-a-boo with baby's hands and feet as you slip them into clothes.

Right: It may take lots of perseverance and patience to convince your baby to wear a hat.

CLOTHING YOUR BABY

Some older babies take an active role in getting dressed, pushing their hand through a sleeve opening or "helping" you pull a jumper off. But if they are not in the mood, dressing can be a challenge. Try to make it as much fun as possible – smile, make eye contact, chat, sing and play games. Clothes that are easy to get on and off make the whole process easier: look for wide necks and sleeves, stretchy fabrics and popper fastenings. If your baby is crawling, choose clothes that keep the knees covered.

A hat is important for warmth in cold weather and to give protection from the sun. But getting a baby to wear one is tricky. If your baby pulls it off as a matter of course, wait until he or she is distracted and then put it back on. Alternatively try saying "No" firmly and replacing it. You may have to do this many times, but once the baby realizes you mean business the hat may stay in place – for a while at least. It will help if the baby has a coat with a hood that you can pull over the hat, or if you choose a hat with straps that fasten under the chin.

Babies don't need shoes until they are walking. Keep the feet bare whenever you are in the warm. If your baby is wearing socks, make sure they are the non-slip variety in the right size: the tiny bones in a baby's feet are very soft, and tight socks can cause damage. Outdoors, a baby's feet may need some extra protection: soft pram shoes are best. Once your child learns to walk, buy proper shoes with lightweight, flexible soles from a specialist shop with trained fitters.

SAFETY IN THE BATH

- The water should be warm but not hot. Always check the temperature before putting the baby in the bath.
- Keep the room warm; babies lose body heat very quickly when they are wet.
- Keep the bath shallow – no more than waist-deep when your baby is sitting down.
- Never leave a baby alone in the bath, or under the care of another child.
- Don't let your baby pull himself or herself up in the bath unless you are holding on. It's best to discourage standing in the bath altogether.
- Wrap a wet facecloth around the hot tap as soon as your baby is old enough to reach for it.
- Put a non-slip mat in the bottom of the bath.

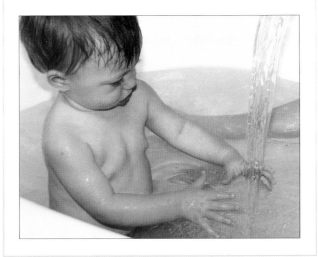

SAFETY IN THE SUN

- Keep your baby out of the sun as much as possible.
- When using a buggy, attach a parasol or, better still, a UV-filter sunshade.
- Dress your baby in lightweight fabric with a tight weave to protect the skin.
- Make your baby wear a wide-brimmed hat.
- Use a sunscreen of factor 20 or above, and re-apply frequently. Choose a natural sun cream specially formulated for children.
- Take precautions on warm cloudy days as well as on sunny ones.

When to wean

By the age of six months, your baby will almost certainly be ready to start eating solid food. The iron stored at birth will have begun to run out, and the baby may need more calories than he or she can get from milk alone. At this age, most babies are interested in new experiences and are more likely to take to eating than if you wait until much later in the first year. Ideally you will start giving solids at six months, but some parents start earlier, and so long as the baby is not at risk of developing allergies and you give only recommended foods, this shouldn't be a problem. However it is important not to start giving your baby food any earlier than four months, because a young baby's intestines are immature. Starting solids early or giving certain foods may encourage long-term digestive problems or allergies.

Young babies also find it quite difficult to eat – which suggests that they are not ready for the experience. They can't sit up properly, so swallowing is difficult, and they tend to poke their tongue out when they sense something alien in their mouths. This tongue-thrust reflex protects them from choking. It disappears between four and six

If your baby shows an interest in food, a bouncy chair is a convenient place to have his or her first meals.

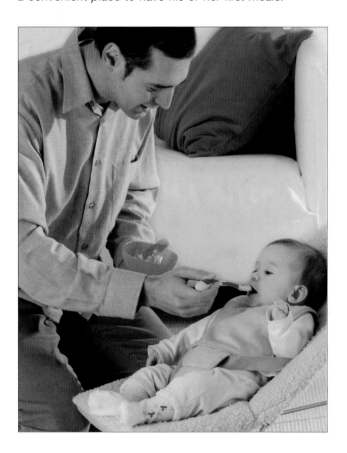

ESSENTIAL EQUIPMENT
You don't need a lot of special equipment when introducing solid food to your baby, but the following are useful.

Baby chair. It is much easier to feed with a spoon when you are facing your baby. If he or she can sit up well, use a highchair. If not, a bouncy chair set at the most upright level makes a good substitute for the first weeks.

Spoons. Shallow weaning spoons are easy to get into a baby's mouth and make it easy for him or her to lick the food off. Plastic spoons are easy to clean and sterilize, and they won't hurt your baby when he or she starts waving them around.

Bibs. Feeding is a messy business so you will need three or more bibs. Cloth ones are the most comfortable, and Velcro fasteners are much easier to use than ties.

Bowls. You can use ordinary bowls, but it is easier to serve tiny amounts in a small, shallow bowl, which also allows the baby to see the food. A bowl with a sucker on the base is good for when a baby starts to feed himself or herself, because it stays steady.

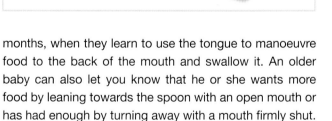

months, when they learn to use the tongue to manoeuvre food to the back of the mouth and swallow it. An older baby can also let you know that he or she wants more food by leaning towards the spoon with an open mouth or has had enough by turning away with a mouth firmly shut.

IS MY BABY READY FOR SOLIDS?
Wait until your baby is showing signs of being interested in food before you think about introducing solids. These are some of the typical signs to look for.
- Your baby still seems hungry after a feed.
- Your baby wants feeding more often.
- Your baby watches you with interest when you eat.
- Your baby begins waking up more frequently in the night after a period of sleeping through.
- Your baby is putting things in his or her mouth.
- Your baby can hold his or her head up well.

Left: Before you use the highchair for feeding, get your baby used to it. Put some toys on the table for them to play with. If they start putting a toy in their mouth, give them something they can eat.

Right: Starting your baby on solids is quite an event. At first it can feel like hard work, but you – and the baby – will soon get the hang of it.

Talk to your health visitor if you are not sure whether to start solids or not. A premature baby won't be ready to start on solids until at least four to six months from his or her expected, rather than actual, birth date.

WHICH HIGHCHAIR?

The most natural option for a highchair is one that is made from wood from a sustainable source. Make sure the design is simple and that it doesn't have any awkward crevices that will be difficult to clean.

A chair with an adjustable seat or footrest will be more comfortable for the baby, but will probably take up more space than one that folds up. The chair should have a fixed five-point harness for absolute safety. You will need some cushioning to protect the baby's head from banging on the back of the chair.

Some highchairs are designed to be drawn up to the table so that the baby can join in family meals from the beginning. This is a great idea in theory, but you may prefer to choose one with a tray to contain the mess. A highchair with a detachable tray can be used either way.

ALLERGIES

If a baby's father, mother or any siblings suffer from allergies or allergy-related conditions such as asthma, eczema or hay fever (allergic rhinitis), the baby may inherit the allergy. The best way to protect him or her is to breastfeed exclusively for six months, and to continue breastfeeding for the rest of the first year.

Introduce solids very slowly and do not give any foods that you or your partner are allergic to until your baby is at least a year old. Dairy foods, wheat, citrus fruits, eggs, fish, shellfish and nuts are the most common food allergens, so they should be introduced with caution. Sesame seeds and peanuts, and any foods containing them (such as peanut butter, groundnut oil and sesame oil) should not be given until your child is at least three; you may wish to exclude all nuts from your child's diet.

Even if there is no family history of allergy, it is still important to take weaning slowly. Introduce one new food at a time and be on the lookout for any allergic reactions. These usually occur within minutes of eating and can include the following: facial rash (especially around the mouth), sneezing, runny nose, coughing, wheezing. Very occasionally, a baby may develop breathing difficulties or swelling of the lips: this needs urgent medical attention and you need to call an ambulance.

If a baby is intolerant of a certain food – meaning it is difficult to digest – he or she may experience bloating or passing wind, diarrhoea or vomiting within a few hours or sometimes over a couple of days after eating it. If your baby seems to have a reaction of this kind to a certain food, try introducing it again a few weeks later to see if the reaction recurs. If it does, you probably need to eliminate the food from your baby's diet. Children often grow out of allergies and intolerances, so you may be able to re-introduce the offending food later, but get individual advice on this from a health professional.

When a baby is ready for weaning, he or she should take food from a spoon or your finger with just a little encouragement.

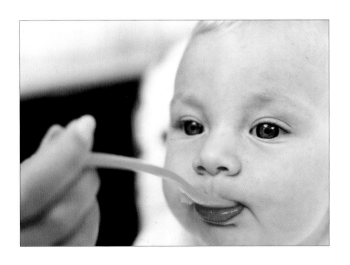

First foods: 4–6 months

Your aim when introducing solids is to get your baby used to different tastes and textures, not to replace milk. Start with just one "meal" a day, offering just a teaspoonful of food to start with. If your baby seems eager for more, you can offer a couple of teaspoonfuls the next time and gradually build up to a couple of tablespoons or so. Don't worry if your baby seems to eat more one day and then less the next; this is quite normal.

A good time to introduce solid food is mid-morning, ideally between milk feeds. That way, your baby won't be so hungry that he or she will be wanting milk, nor so full that he or she won't be interested in trying something new. Once the baby is used to the idea, you can combine solid food with the lunchtime feed. Give milk before the solids, so that you don't cut down on milk feeds too quickly. Or try giving a little milk first, then the solids, then the rest of the milk.

If your baby rejects the food repeatedly, he or she probably isn't ready for solids yet and you should wait a week or two before trying again. Don't try to force the baby to eat more than he or she wants – babies have a good sense of when to stop and it is important to be led by what your baby wants.

Avocado and banana, mashed together, are healthy raw foods that you can feed to young babies.

INTRODUCING NEW TASTES

Give baby rice for at least a week or two before introducing another new food. Take the weaning process very slowly, introducing new foods one a time. Leave about a week between the first three or four new foods

Starting solids

A good first food is baby rice, which is gluten-free and unlikely to cause any reaction. Commercial baby rice comes in dried flakes and usually has added nutrients such as iron. Mix it with your baby's usual milk (expressed breastmilk or formula) so that this first "meal" has a familiar taste. It should have a soupy consistency.

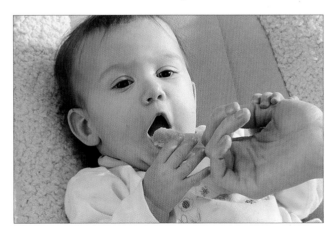

1 Put a little of the milky baby rice on the tip of your finger so that your baby can suck it off. If he or she doesn't seem interested, try dabbing a little on his or her lips or tongue. You may find that the rice is poked straight back out until your baby gets the hang of moving it to the back of the mouth for swallowing.

2 If your baby takes well to sucking food off your finger, offer a little rice on a shallow spoon. Give a few more spoonfuls if the baby shows interest by leaning forwards, opening his or her mouth when you offer the food, or grabbing your finger or the spoon. If the baby turns away or pushes your hand away, he or she has had enough.

and wait three to five days before introducing subsequent ones. This will allow your baby's digestive system to get used to each new food, and will also make it easier for you to pinpoint the problem food if your baby develops an allergic reaction.

The following fruits and vegetables make excellent first foods because they are bland and can be mashed or puréed to a smooth consistency. Add a little milk or milky baby rice so that the consistency is fairly runny. To make food more interesting, combine different purées that you have already introduced – try carrot and apple, parsnip and sweet potato, papaya and banana.

Root vegetables. These have a naturally sweet taste and are easy to digest. Try carrots, sweet potato, butternut squash, yams, parsnips and swede (rutabaga). Peel and cut into pieces (remove the seeds in squash), steam until very soft and then purée or mash. Your baby may also like puréed potato.

The best way to cook fruits and vegetables for babies is to steam them – it preserves more nutrients than any other cooking method.

Pears and apples. These fruits are gentle on the stomach and most babies love them. Peel, core and cut into pieces. Steam or cook in a little water until very soft, then purée or mash. An older baby can eat mashed, uncooked pear if it is very ripe.

Bananas, papayas and avocados. These are very digestible fruits that don't need cooking. Simply mash and mix with a little milk to give a suitably runny texture.

COOKING FOR A BABY

The best cooking method is steaming, which preserves most nutrients. Boiling and baking (without oil) are also healthy, but don't boil foods for too long. Avoid frying and roasting, which makes food more difficult to digest. Microwaving not only destroys some of the nutrients in food, but also heats it unevenly, so it is best avoided.

To save time, you can cook and purée a batch of vegetables or fruit, take what you need for one meal, cool the rest and freeze straight away in ice-cube trays. When the cubes are frozen, transfer them to a freezer bag. Don't forget to date and label the bag. Cooked frozen foods cannot be refrozen once defrosted, and if your baby does not eat much of a meal you must throw the rest away, however wasteful that seems. It is fine to defrost frozen food cubes in a saucepan, but make sure that you heat the food through thoroughly, then cool before feeding.

THREE MEALS A DAY

A few weeks after you start giving your baby solids mid-morning, you can introduce breakfast, too. Most babies are very hungry when they wake up, so give a milk feed first and then a teaspoon or two of solids. After another few weeks, start giving the baby some solids in the early evening, too. You can gradually increase the amount at each meal to suit his or her appetite – follow your baby's lead and give what he or she seems to want. Older babies will also need healthy snacks between meals, such as fruit, rice cakes and oatcakes.

The best way to cook fruits and vegetables for babies is to steam them – it preserves more nutrients than any other cooking method.

Preparing a batch of tiny meals in advance takes the stress out of feeding.

Baby rice is quick and easy to prepare, and most babies like it.

Second foods: 6–8 months

Once you have introduced the idea of eating solid food, the next step is to extend your baby's palate. Don't assume that your baby won't like strong flavours such as, say, courgette (zucchini) or natural yoghurt; he or she may well surprise you. It will help if you introduce each new food in a relaxed and confident way – if your expression says "Beware", then your child will. Often a baby will be more willing to accept a new food that has a distinctive flavour – spinach, say – if it is mixed with the carrot or parsnip that he or she already knows and loves. Start by adding a tiny amount and then gradually increase the ratio of spinach to carrot as the baby gets used to it.

NEW FOODS TO TRY

The following foods are good ones to introduce after the first, rather bland, foods. Remember to introduce them one at a time, and to leave three to five days between each new food.

FOODS THAT NEED TO WAIT
Some foods are more likely to cause an allergic reaction than others, so they should not be among the first foods that you introduce to your baby.

After six months, you can give:
- Cow's milk dairy products – yoghurts, butter, cheese and fromage frais, but don't give unpasteurized cheeses to a young child.

After eight months, you can give:
- Foods containing gluten – wheat, rye, barley or oats
- Egg yolk (make sure it is well cooked)
- Nuts and seeds that have been ground (excluding peanuts and sesame seeds)
- Fish (but children should not have shark, marlin or swordfish because they contain levels of mercury that could affect their developing nervous systems)
- Citrus fruits and juices.

After twelve months, you can give:
- Honey (avoid for the first year because it may contain a bacterium that causes infant botulism)
- Peanuts (crushed) and sesame seeds (avoid until three years if there is a family history of nut allergy)
- Nuts that have been chopped (whole nuts should not be given to a child under five years because of the risk of choking).

CAUTION
Never leave your baby alone when eating: stay nearby in case he or she chokes on a piece of food.

Vegetables. Try purées of steamed courgette, spinach or green beans, broccoli and cauliflower, as well as puréed boiled frozen peas. Home-cooked beetroot (beet) is a good food to combine with mashed potato.

Fruits. Lightly cooked mangoes, peaches and nectarines make good purées, or try mashed ripe melon (cantaloupe is one of the sweetest) from about seven months. Dried fruits such as apricots, dates or prunes can be cooked in water and then puréed, but give them sparingly as they are very sweet. Some babies are allergic to kiwi fruit and strawberries, so wait until at least nine months before introducing these fruits and watch for any reaction.

Grains. Introduce millet or oats (which can be made into a smooth porridge) before wheat-based cereals, which are more likely to cause a reaction. Once your baby is taking textured food, couscous, quinoa and barley are good grain foods and you can also introduce tiny pasta shapes (buy the ones intended for soup).

Dairy products. Give plain unsweetened yoghurt, plain

Babies have a natural instinct to do things for themselves, and most really enjoy feeding themselves with finger foods. Rice cakes are ideal to start off with because they disintegrate when sucked.

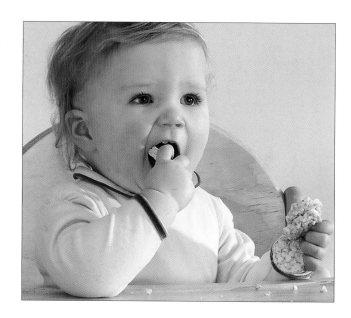

fromage frais, cream cheese, cottage cheese, Cheddar and other hard cheeses. Always use full-fat dairy products – growing babies need lots of calories so you don't want them to fill up on low-fat foods.

Lentils and beans. Try a purée of red lentils – you can add a sliver each of garlic and ginger to the cooking water to add flavour (remove the ginger before puréeing). From about nine months you can try butterbeans, haricots, split peas and soya.

Chicken and meat. Chicken and turkey usually go down well. They can be puréed or mashed with root or green vegetables or dairy products. Once your baby is happy with white meat try lean red meat such as lamb.

Fish. Introduce white fish from about eight months: poach it in milk, flake it and check very carefully for bones before feeding to your baby. Once your baby is happily eating these foods, you can try introducing oily fish such as salmon.

EXTRA FLAVOURS

You can make your baby's food more tasty by adding flavourings such as sautéed onion or leek, garlic and ginger, and finely chopped parsley and other soft-leaved herbs. It is also a good idea to introduce mild spices from about eight months – try sprinkling a little cinnamon on porridge, or adding cumin or paprika to savoury dishes.

Don't add any salt to food for a baby less than a year old, and avoid processed foods such as baked beans, which contain added salt. Similarly, don't sweeten food with sugar or give sugary "treats". There can be a lot of

Introduce your baby to different textures and tastes. Try a whole banana, oatcakes, a few raisins or dried apricots, a handful of whole butter (lima) beans, chunks of hard cheese, thin slices of apple or pear and tiny sandwich squares spread with cream cheese.

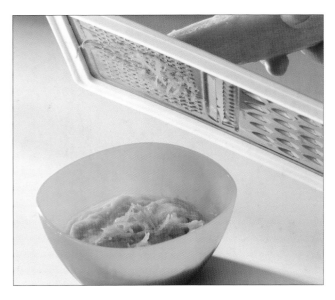

Adding grated food to purées is a good way of getting your baby used to a new texture.

sugar in fruity yoghurts and fromage frais, baby rusks and processed foods, and all are best avoided.

TEXTURE, TOO

At first your baby can manage only smooth and runny purées. But if you go on giving these for a long time, he or she may reject lumpier food. So it is a good idea to start mashing rather than puréeing food from about seven months, and to gradually increase the lumpiness of the food you serve. Once your baby is eating lumpier food, try stirring in some finely grated or chopped foods to introduce different textures. You can also give your baby finger foods from about seven months.

Don't limit your baby to bland foods. Babies are much more receptive to new flavours than older children, so it is a good idea to expose them to flavours such as ginger, cumin, garlic and fresh herbs.

Healthy eating for babies

As your baby's appetite for solid food increases over the first year, he or she will start to take less milk. Once solids become a more substantial part of the diet, you need to start providing a good mix of different foods to ensure that your baby is getting all the right nutrients. A balanced daily diet for a nine- to twelve-month-old baby would include the following.

One or two servings of protein foods. Protein is made up of amino acids, which are needed for the growth and repair of all the body's cells and tissues. Lean meat, chicken and turkey, fish, eggs, cheese, yoghurt and tofu (soya bean curd) are complete sources of protein. Pulses and beans are healthy protein foods but contain only some of the essential amino acids. Your baby also needs to eat some grain foods (rice, oats, bread or pasta) or nuts and seeds over the course of the day to get a good balance of amino acids.

Three or four servings of starchy foods. Carbohydrates are the body's main fuel. The best sources are starchy foods such as oats, rice, bread, barley, rye and potatoes; lentils, pulses, fruits and vegetables also contain carbohydrates. It is best not to feed babies high-fibre foods as this will fill their tiny stomachs without providing the necessary nutrients. Refined grains such as white rice and ordinary pasta are much easier to digest.

Four or five servings of fruits and vegetables. These contain the vitamins and minerals that are essential to good health, and they are the best source of fibre for babies and young children. The best way to make sure that your baby is getting enough is to offer as wide a range as possible.

Grains and starchy vegetables give your baby the carbohydrates he or she needs for energy.

Cheese, yoghurt and other dairy foods are a good source of calcium, but be sure to give full-fat versions.

Calcium. Babies get calcium from their milk, which is still their most important food. If your baby is not drinking quite enough milk, other good dietary sources include dairy products (cheese, yoghurt, fromage frais), almonds, brazil nuts, green leafy vegetables and tofu.

Some healthy fats. Fats are a concentrated source of calories, which growing babies need – both breastmilk and formula have high fat contents. Always give your baby full-fat versions of any milk, cheese, yoghurt or other dairy products you offer. Include healthy

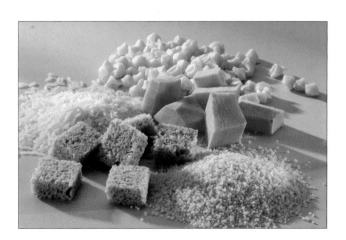

GOING ORGANIC

Buying organic food is an easy way to reduce the chemicals your baby is exposed to: organic fruits and vegetables are produced with fewer pesticides and fertilizers, and the animals used for organic meat are not routinely given antibiotics. Organic farming methods may also produce some food with higher levels of nutrients: one study found that organic milk had higher levels of essential fatty acids, vitamin E and antioxidants, which help fight infection.

PACKED WITH VITAMINS

Vitamin	Needed for	Good sources
Vitamin A	Growth, healthy skin, good eyesight	Green leafy vegetables, carrots, squash, sweet potatoes, apricots, mangoes, liver, oily fish, egg yolks, butter, margarine and cheese
Vitamin B group	Growth, healthy nervous and immune systems, healthy skin, nails and hair, good digestion	Green leafy vegetables, broccoli, oats, lean meat and liver, tofu, fish, fortified breakfast cereals, bananas, avocados, milk and yoghurt
Vitamin C	Strong gums, teeth, bones and skin, healthy immune system, helps with iron absorption	Citrus and berry fruits, mangoes, papaya, nectarines, blackcurrants, potatoes, green leafy vegetables, peppers, tomatoes
Vitamin D	Strong bones and teeth	Salmon, sardines, tuna, milk, fortified margarine, eggs, fortified breakfast cereals
Vitamin E	Maintaining the body's cell structure	Vegetable oils, nuts, seeds, avocado

unsaturated fats in the baby's diet, from vegetable oils, avocados, nuts and seeds, and oily fish. Foods such as processed cakes and crisps contain unhealthy trans-fats and have no nutritional value so they should be avoided altogether.

Some iron-rich foods. Iron is important both for physical and for mental growth, but babies can easily become anaemic (iron-deficient). Use a formula milk with extra iron if you are bottle-feeding. Good dietary sources of iron include red meat and liver, oily fish, pulses, green leafy vegetables, dried fruits such as apricots, and fortified breakfast cereals. Iron from animal sources is easily absorbed by the body. Iron from plant-based sources is absorbed more easily if they are accompanied by a food that is rich in vitamin C (red (bell) peppers, tomatoes and all citrus fruits are particularly good).

Protein foods such as meat, fish, lentils and eggs are an important part of a baby's diet.

Try to get your baby to try different kinds of fresh fruits, to provide a good range of vitamins.

VEGETARIAN BABIES

A vegetarian diet is perfectly healthy for babies so long as they get enough protein: offer two servings a day. An easy way to increase the protein content of a vegetarian meal is to add cheese, chopped egg yolk or a smooth cashew or almond nut butter (from about eight months). You'll also need to ensure that a vegetarian baby gets sufficient iron, especially if still being breastfed (formula has added iron), and vitamin B12, found in dairy products, breakfast cereals and yeast extract (suitable after one year).

A vegan diet is very restrictive, so it is harder to make sure your baby is getting all the necessary nutrients. You'll have to plan meals carefully in order to provide the baby with enough protein, vitamin B12 and vitamin D, and you may need to give vitamin supplements. It is worth getting advice from a paediatric dietician or doctor before starting to wean your baby if you intend to follow a vegan diet.

Milk and the older baby

Babies need to continue drinking plenty of milk, even after solids are introduced. They need about 600ml/1 pint a day up to the age of twelve months. Give your baby milk first thing in the morning and at bedtime, and at other times if necessary.

Breastmilk is the best milk for your baby for the first year. If you are breastfeeding, it is impossible to tell how much milk your baby is getting. But if you are giving four or more full feeds a day, your baby is almost certainly getting enough.

Bottle-fed babies over the age of six months can continue to drink infant formula or can switch to a follow-on milk if the infant formula doesn't seem to be satisfying them. Cow's milk and goat's milk are not suitable as a main drink until your baby is at least twelve months old, because they don't have enough iron and other nutrients.

OTHER DRINKS

Other than milk, the best drink to give is water. There's no need to give other drinks, which fill your baby up without providing vital calories. It is a good idea to get your child used to drinking water from an early age. Give him or her sips from a cup at mealtimes.

Babies over the age of six months can drink water straight from the tap, but you may want to filter it first to remove impurities. Don't give bottled mineral water – some have high levels of salt and are unsuitable for babies, and the water may have been sitting in the bottle for months.

A spouted cup is useful when you are out and about, and there is a wide range on the market – you may need to experiment to find one your baby likes to use. Remember it is still important to sterilize your baby's cups, bottles and teats.

Mother's milk is still the best nutrition a baby can have – it has a high fat content to give energy and plenty of calcium for growing bones.

Fruit juice, even if it is well diluted, is too acidic for young babies. Even after six months, it is best not to give your baby fruit juice to drink because it contains sugars, which can cause tooth decay. Sometimes parents are advised to give babies diluted juice at mealtimes to help

Weaning your baby off a bottle and on to a cup can be a long process. Try cuddling your baby in the same way you would when they were taking a bottle, and maintaining the close association milk has with you.

Left: There's no need to give your baby sweet fruity yoghurts. Try him or her on plain bio-active yoghurt, which is better for the teeth and can help the digestion.

Right: Dairy foods, such as milk, cheese and yoghurt, are a good way of ensuring that babies get enough calcium in their diet.

them absorb the iron in food. But fruit or vegetables rich in vitamin C will do the job just as well. If you do decide to give juice at mealtimes, dilute it with water – ten parts water to one part juice – to help protect your baby's emerging teeth, and to stop them getting full on liquid. Other drinks, such as squashes, teas or fizzy drinks, should never be given to a baby.

MOVING TO A CUP

It's a good idea to start getting your baby used to a cup from six or seven months. With a bottle, liquid tends to collect in the mouth and over a prolonged period this can lead to tooth decay, particularly if the baby tends to comfort suck. Frequent sucking on a teat can also interfere with the correct development of a baby's teeth.

The best kind of cup to use is an open one; you can get slanted "Doidy" cups, which are easier for a baby to drink from than the usual baby cup with a spout. You are bound to have accidents when using an open cup, so you may want to restrict it to times when your baby is sitting on your lap or in a highchair and use a beaker with a spout (a sippy cup) for water at other times.

It can take a long time to get a bottle-fed baby used to drinking from a cup. Take your time – and don't be surprised if it takes six months or more to completely wean the baby from a bottle. The bedtime bottle is usually the last one to go, but don't worry, just enjoy the warmth and closeness it brings. Here are some ways to help.

- Let the baby play with an empty cup.
- Introduce a cup at mealtimes first, and help your baby to hold it.
- When you think your baby is ready, give one milk feed from a cup. Choose a feed when the baby doesn't drink as much – usually the mid-afternoon one.
- Keep your baby cuddled on your lap while he or she is drinking the milk – some babies are reluctant to give up the bottle because they associate it with being held.
- Once your baby is taking the cup at one feed, substitute it for the bottle at other feeds, one at a time.

WEANING FROM THE BREAST

The decision to wean your baby from the breast is a complicated and emotive one. Babies benefit from having breastmilk as their main drink throughout the first year, but many nursing women decide that they want to stop or reduce breastfeeds earlier for a variety of good reasons.

- Don't stop breastfeeding abruptly, since this can be traumatic for your baby and uncomfortable for you.
- Accept that weaning takes time. Leave at least a week or two between each dropping of a feed.
- Substitute a bottle or cup of milk for each feed you drop so that your baby doesn't go short of milk.
- If the baby is reluctant, try giving expressed breastmilk until he or she gets used to the idea of taking milk from a source other than the breast.
- If your baby won't take a bottle or cup from you, then try getting his or her father to give it. Stay out of the room so that you don't distract the baby.
- Give your baby lots of cuddles. It is important that he or she doesn't feel rejected and continues to get the closeness you both enjoy when you breastfeed.
- Make the bedtime feed the last one you drop. You may decide that you are happy to continue with this, and a morning feed, say, for a few months longer if your baby is drinking formula at other times.
- Wear a well-fitting bra. Express a little milk to prevent engorgement if necessary.

SUPPLEMENTS FOR BREASTFED BABIES

While breastmilk is generally healthier than formula milk, formula does have iron and vitamins added to it. Breast-fed babies may not get enough vitamin A, C and D from milk alone, so vitamin drops are generally advised. However, once they start eating solids, babies can get these vitamins from other foods; vitamin D is also made by the body when the skin is exposed to sunlight.

Helping your baby enjoy food

Eating is one of life's great joys. It's common for parents to worry about how much and what their baby is eating, but such anxiety can introduce an element of tension into mealtimes that is counterproductive. Having a relaxed, positive attitude towards your baby's food will go a long way to helping him or her enjoy it.

MAKING FOOD FUN

Let your baby eat with his or her fingers. Food will go all over the place, but it will show that eating is fun and that the baby can feed himself or herself rather than having to rely on you to spoon food into his or her mouth. Once old enough, your baby will love to pick up peas or other small morsels and pop them into his or her mouth. Serve easy finger foods alongside mashed or minced food – try steamed strips of vegetables, thin strips of chicken, strips of rolled-up pancakes, butter (lima) beans, small pasta shapes and squares of toast.

Give your baby a spoon as soon as he or she wants to hold one. Let the baby try to use it, while you use a second spoon to get food into his or her mouth, and accept the fact that babies make a mess at mealtimes. Don't hover around wiping your baby's face or hands after

Your baby may assert a fierce sense of independence at mealtimes. Feeding will probably work best at this stage if you both have a spoon.

every mouthful – you'll be sending out the message that food is dirty or bad. Use a bib and put newspaper or a plastic sheet under the highchair to contain the mess. Wait until mealtime is over to clean the baby up.

RELAXED MEALTIMES

Always sit with your baby when he or she eats: mealtimes should be sociable events, and you need to stay close by in case of choking. Include the baby in family meals from as young an age as possible. Offer suitable bits and pieces off your plate, feed the baby a minced or mashed version of what you are eating or provide some finger foods to play with.

Always be positive about your baby's food. Be careful if you are offering something that you personally don't like – your baby may pick up on your distaste and refuse it. And get into good habits yourself. Your child is more likely to eat fruit at breakfast, say, if he or she sees you doing the same.

Let your baby decide how much to eat. His or her appetite will vary from day to day, and from meal to meal. Don't force food into the baby's mouth or spend ages trying to encourage him or her to eat one last spoonful. Your baby will quickly realize that it's possible to get your focused attention by refusing food, and mealtimes could become a battleground.

Setting a good example

Eating food from the same plate as your baby is a good way of encouraging him or her to eat.

1 If your baby seems uncertain about trying a new food, try popping a bit in your own mouth. Look as though you are enjoying it, and your baby will love to copy you.

2 The next stage will be them wanting to feed you. Accept their offering, however sucked and squishy it might be. They will automatically pick up this positive attitude.

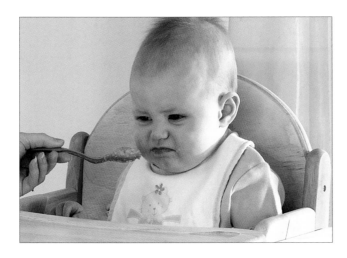

If your baby refuses food, don't keep pushing him or her to accept it – it's more important that the baby sees food as pleasurable than that he or she eats up that last bit of carrot.

EXCITING FLAVOURS

Give homemade food most or all of the time. Most commercial baby foods have a similar taste and they are all processed to the same smoothness. So a baby fed mostly from jars won't experience the distinct flavours and different textures of homemade foods. If you limit your baby to just a few dishes, he or she may be less willing to accept new foods later on, so provide lots of variety. Now is the time to get the baby enjoying as many of the wonderful flavours of food as possible.

REFUSING SOLIDS

Some babies do not take to solids well. If your baby doesn't seem interested when you first offer them, he or she may not be ready for food. Trying waiting at least a week or two before offering it again.

Even babies who take well to solid food will refuse it from time to time, especially if they are ill or teething. The best way to handle this is to stay calm. Continue to offer meals, but leave it up to your baby whether or not he or she eats. Most babies will start eating again when they feel ready, though it can take a few weeks before their appetite returns fully. Similarly, babies will often eat only a few foods – fruit and toast, say – or suddenly refuse foods that they have previously enjoyed. Again, this is normal. Keep offering other foods alongside the ones your baby is eating; let the baby see you eating them. It may also help if you give the baby meals with the rest of the family. Eventually curiousity about new foods will grow again.

WHEN BABIES DON'T EAT

A few babies don't take to eating until much later in the first year. So long as your baby is gaining weight and is healthy, starting solids later is unlikely to be a problem. Talk to a health professional if you are worried. If your

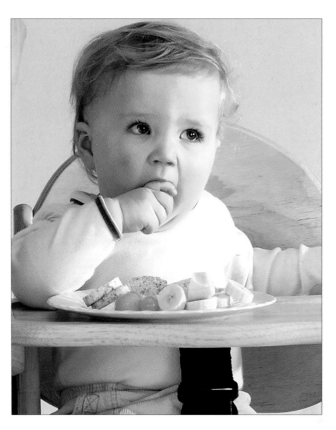

Giving your child a selection of fruit such as grapes and sliced banana after a meal is just as nice – and a lot healthier – than a sugary pudding.

baby is older than eight months and still showing no interest, try cutting down on milk feeds – babies don't need more than 600ml/1 pint per day.

It is worth bearing in mind that a baby who is prone to allergies may be better off feeding only on breastmilk for most of the first year. Nutritionally, babies can get almost everything they need from breastmilk, with the possible exception of iron. Breastmilk contains small amounts of iron, but it is more easily absorbed than that in infant formula, so a breastfed baby may be getting enough.

Your baby will enjoy mealtimes more if he or she is allowed to touch, squash and smear food around. This helps babies to get familiar with food and appreciate it.

Crying, comfort and sleeping

> " Of course, some broken nights are inevitable. They are an inalienable facet of parenthood, well into the toddler years. "

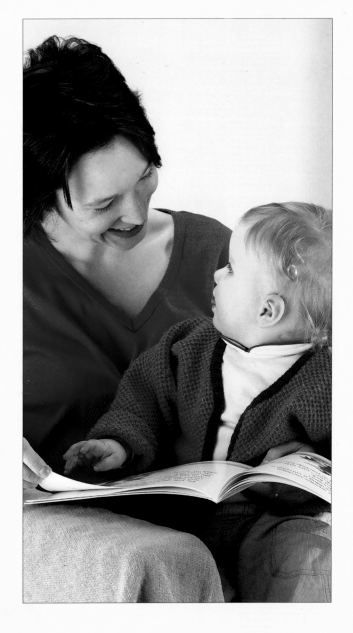

As your baby grows older, you will probably find that he or she cries less frequently. Some of the things that used to be upsetting might now be amusing instead. And while the discomfort of, say, a wet nappy will still trouble a baby, crying will often cease as soon as he or she knows you are attending to the problem. Sometimes your child will just whimper to let you know that something is wrong. In short, your baby has understood that crying is a form of communication, but you still need to respond quickly and compassionately. This can get harder from about eight months, when your baby's intense attachment to you means that he or she may wail in despair if you leave the room. This fear of abandonment, known as separation anxiety, can be very trying for you. When your baby demands to be with you every second, even a simple household task such as boiling the kettle becomes difficult. But the more gently and lovingly you respond to your baby's feelings, the better: he or she needs reassurance to get through this tricky stage.

The bond between parent and child grows stronger in the second six months – and your baby may not want to let you out of his or her sight for a while.

Dealing with nighttime crying is a tougher problem to solve, because you need your baby to spend the nights without your presence. Even babies who have been sleeping well begin to object to going to bed at this age, and no baby likes to wake up in the small hours and find that he or she is alone in the room.

Most babies need guidance to help them sleep well by themselves. This chapter suggests some ways to help your baby to wind down at the end of the day, and how to set clear and consistent rules about bedtime. These techniques will improve a wakeful baby's nights, but to make them work you need to make a clear decision about how you want your baby to sleep, and you must plan to achieve it. Of course, some broken nights are inevitable. They are an inalienable facet of parenthood, well into the toddler years.

Top: Adopt a bedtime routine that stays the same each evening and gives time for your baby to settle down and relax. This will help him or her to fall happily asleep.

With a little forethought and determination, you and your baby can look forward to a refreshing night's sleep more often than not.

Why your baby cries

Older babies cry for many of the same reasons as younger ones: hunger, fear, teething and so on. Older babies cry when they are tired, but don't realize what they need is to go to sleep: unlike young babies they can, and do, keep themselves awake. Good daytime and nighttime sleep routines will help to avoid this problem.

There are also a few new causes for tears, arising from babies' increasing activity and growing perceptions of their world. As your baby learns to crawl, pull up to standing and cruise around the furniture, there are bound to be a few bumps. Crying is more likely to be caused by the shock than any pain, but he or she needs your reassuring hug fast. Older babies also need more stimulation and may cry from boredom: gone are the days when you could walk around shops with the pram for hours at a time. Your baby may quickly get fed up with being confined, and probably has a new moan or whining cry to signal displeasure.

Older babies may scream with fury when things don't happen the way they want. They hate it when they cannot quite make a toy work or find that they are propelling themselves backwards when they are trying to crawl forwards. This sense of frustration isn't necessarily a bad

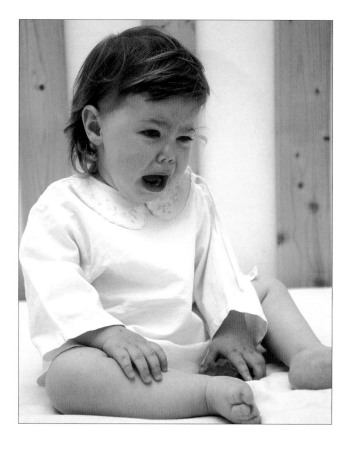

Babies have intense emotions, but unhappiness doesn't last long if they are given comfort or distraction. Older babies are quite capable of crying simply from boredom and lack of stimulation.

Don't leave a baby crying in their cot unless you are following a controlled crying routine. If a baby is crying they are calling for your care and attention, they are not being "naughty".

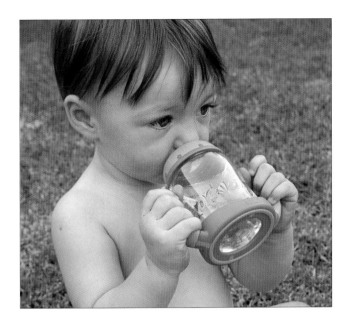

Try not to get into the habit of offering your baby something to eat to stop him or her crying – a few sips of water or an interesting toy will do just as well, and will avoid creating a link between comfort and eating.

thing. It eggs babies on to new achievements, and the screams that accompany their attempts are sometimes a way of expressing the effort they are putting in, but you will obviously want to reduce and minimize any distress.

Help your baby out by showing how to make that troublesome toy work or by removing an obstacle in his or her path. But don't take over – encourage the baby to have another go if the task is within his or her capability. Distraction is the subtlest tool that a parent can deploy. If your baby is getting very frustrated, divert his or her attention by doing something unusual, like making a funny face or a new noise. Remain calm yourself. Cries of frustration are a normal and inevitable part of your baby's development, and patience and reassurance are sometimes all a parent can offer.

THE START OF DISCIPLINE

Lots of people talk about babies being manipulative when they cry. It is true that once a baby learns that you will come running when you hear crying, he or she may do it simply to get your company. But this doesn't make the baby "naughty" or "cunning"– it simply means that he or she wants you to be there. The fact that the crying stops as soon as you arrive shows how delighted your child is to see you.

The next few months, though, are the time to lay the foundations of discipline. As the baby learns to assert himself or herself, you are bound to find that your wishes conflict. For example, your child may scream and resist whenever you try to put him or her in a car seat, or howl in protest when you take that sharp pencil away. Try not to forbid your baby to do things if there is no need. Going

CAUTION
Remember that unexplained crying can be a sign of illness; do see your doctor if you feel worried or if your baby has any unusual symptoms.

into the car seat is obviously non-negotiable, but perhaps it doesn't matter if the baby pulls all the food containers out of the cupboard: this is only exploring after all, and your baby doesn't know that they are not toys. So choose your battles wisely: it will make life easier for you both.

Be firm. If you have decided that your baby cannot do something – such as playing with your mobile phone – don't suddenly give in.

Be consistent. Don't stop your baby pulling books off a shelf one day and then ignore this same behaviour the very next day.

Be inventive. If your baby is resisting going into the highchair, say, put an exciting object on the tray to encourage him or her to go willingly.

Think prevention. You can avoid a lot of tears by ensuring your baby's environment is safe to explore.

Reinforce words with action. Don't expect your baby to stop doing something because you call "No" from the other side of the room without moving towards them; it is good to say "No" in a firm way but you should also go and gently take the troublesome object away to reinforce the message. Add some easily understood words of explanation as well – for example, "Hot!" as you move the baby away from the oven.

If a child is crying from anger or frustration try to keep calm yourself, and keep giving love and cuddles.

Fear and anxiety

There is a whole category of things that can make your baby cry that are nothing to do with the physical world but are psychological in nature. By now your baby has built up an expectation of how things happen in his or her world. If something out of the ordinary happens – even if it is not a bad thing in itself – the baby may cry because it is unsettling. For example, if you take your child to a swimming pool for the first time, he or she may cry even before you go into the water, because the smell, look and sound of the pool environment are very unfamiliar. Similarly, if a babysitter appears when the baby wakes in the night, instead of you or your partner, he or she may become very distressed – even if the babysitter is somebody your baby loves.

The best way to help your baby through these difficulties is to try to let him or her know whenever something new is about to happen. The babysitter could call to your baby while approaching the room, so that the baby knows someone different is coming in before he or

Fathers need not be upset if their baby cries when handed over. Babies naturally feel closest to their mother at first: the uniquely wonderful and complex bond with the father takes longer to develop.

she is picked up and comforted. And, of course, your baby will be much easier to soothe if left in the care of someone he or she knows well. At the swimming pool, cuddle the baby for a while and point out other children playing in the water before you even attempt to get in there too. Babies are very adaptable and usually enjoy new experiences, so long as they are introduced gradually and from a home base of safety.

FEARS

Older babies may develop very specific fears of everyday things. A classic one is the vacuum cleaner. Even if you used the sound of a vacuum cleaner to lull your newborn to sleep, you may find that an older baby develops a real fear of it. This may be so great that the baby whimpers on catching a glimpse and cries at a similar sound – such as the blender, say, or a hedge trimmer being used outside.

Although your baby's fears may seem irrational, don't dismiss them as "silly" or try to force him or her to confront them – you will only increase the fear. Babies need to feel safe in the world and to know that they can trust their carers to look after them. So if your baby is scared of the vacuum cleaner, keep it out of sight and use it only when he or she is sleeping or in another room. If the baby seems to be scared of the dark, get a nightlight or leave the hall light on and the bedroom door open.

As your baby is reassured about being protected from frightening things, his or her confidence will grow. Eventually the baby may start to get curious about the very thing that was scary – he or she may want to look at that vacuum cleaner and even touch it. Don't rush this – let the baby conquer such fears one step at a time, when he or she is ready.

SEPARATION ANXIETY

Young babies think of themselves and their main carers as one: they have no sense of themselves as individuals and are completely unaware that those tiny fists waving in the air belong to them. As they learn to control their movements and make things happen, they gradually become aware that they are independent beings. One clue is the realization that they can make the carer come by crying out, which happens at about four months.

By about seven months, they have worked out that they and their carers are separate entities. This marks a huge leap in understanding, but it also makes babies anxious: for if they are separate, that means they can be left alone. Separation anxiety, as it is known, manifests as

Left: It is amazing how the most heartbreaking tears can be soothed and then forgotten by a live-in-the-moment toddler.

Right: If you are leaving your child, be sure to say a proper goodbye that isn't rushed or stressful. Sneaking off may avoid some tears at the time but it will make him or her feel insecure.

a tendency to cling. It usually starts between eight and twelve months; but it can be later and some babies are not affected at all.

Your baby may start to cry if you try to give him or her to other people, especially if they are not very familiar. The baby may also protest or burst into tears if you leave the room for a moment, even when being cuddled by the grandfather he or she loves. At this stage, your baby cannot understand that you will return – all he or she feels is abandonment.

All the effort you put into your baby's feelings of security and confidence in the early years helps them as they get older and spend more time without you.

HANDLING SEPARATION ANXIETY

Your baby needs to be secure in his or her attachment to you. Only through love and reassurance do babies gain the confidence to explore the world.

Keep your baby with you as much as possible. It is often easier to take the baby with you into the bathroom, say, than to cause unnecessary distress. If your baby becomes nervous of strangers, which is very common during the second half-year, don't pass him or her over for a cuddle. Ignore anyone who says he or she is spoiled or clingy; your child will go to other people when he or she is good and ready. If possible, however, get your baby used to being with at least one other trusted person beside you and your partner. This means that there is someone else to care for him or her in an emergency, or if you really need a break.

When you are leaving, always say goodbye – sneaking off when your baby's attention is distracted for a moment will undermine his or her trust in you. But keep goodbyes short, cheery and calm – if you show that you are upset or anxious, you will be reaffirming and increasing the baby's sense of unease. It's a good idea to use the same form of words (perhaps with an accompanying gesture) each time. For example, say "One minute" (and hold up one finger) if you are just popping into another room to get something; say "See you later" (and blow a kiss) if you will be away for longer. And if you have said you will be "one minute", don't be gone for ages – always stick to your promises. Your baby doesn't understand the concept of time yet, but will come to realize that "one minute" means a short separation.

Give your full attention to your baby when you get back. Have a loving cuddle straight away if the baby wants one; if he or she is happily absorbed in doing something, watch and perhaps join in until your baby is ready to come to you. Be cheerful but calm so that the baby learns your return is quite normal and not something to make a big fuss about. Gradually your baby will learn that you always come back.

Changing sleep patterns

By now your baby will almost certainly be sleeping a lot more at night than in the day. Babies over six months commonly sleep for ten to twelve hours at night, as well as having daytime naps. But your nights are still unlikely to be the long unbroken stretch you may be craving. Even though your baby may be sleeping for as much as six to eight hours at a time, the longest sleep will probably coincide with your evening and the early part of your night. Most babies wake up at least once a night until they are twelve months old.

It is still important to put older babies on their back to sleep. If you find that your baby rolls over, gently move him or her back again. However, if this happens repeatedly or if the baby wakes up when turned, it is probably better to leave him or her be.

DAYTIME NAPS

Most babies need at least two naps a day – one in the morning and one in the early afternoon – until the end of the first year. Ideally, the afternoon nap should be the long one, as it will help keep your baby going until bedtime.

Some babies drop a nap even before they get to twelve months. You might find that they just enjoy a quiet period at that time for a couple of weeks.

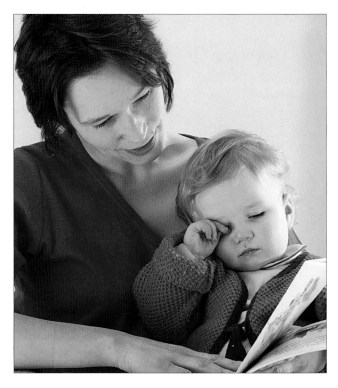

Your baby may be happy to play with some toys in the cot even if he or she doesn't want a nap. If not, schedule in some quiet time – look at a book or do a simple jigsaw – as a break in an action-packed day.

Now that your baby is more aware of what is going on, he or she may resist going to sleep during the day, because who wants to nap when there is all that exploring to do? But rest is important, otherwise the baby will become irritable during the day and, paradoxically, will find it harder to sleep at night.

Do what you can to facilitate naps, whether this means putting the baby down in a darkened room or rocking him or her to sleep in a buggy. If possible, put your baby down soon after lunch, even if there is no sign of tiredness. Without a sleep in the early afternoon, he or she is likely to be exhausted by late afternoon, the worst time for a nap because bedtime is not far away.

Don't worry too much about how long your baby sleeps. Although the average baby naps for about three hours a day, yours may need a lot less sleep than this. Be guided by your baby's humour and habits – if he or she is in a good mood during the day and sleeps well at night, then it doesn't matter if the naps are very short.

Some babies drop a nap before they reach twelve months. Usually the morning nap is the first to go, but some drop their afternoon nap, which means they have a

Moving your baby to his or her own room may improve the nights for all of you. The baby may be more inclined to settle him or herself after waking at night.

long time awake before bedtime. One solution might be to give your baby an early lunch – 11 am, say – and to put him or her down for a nap after that.

BABY'S OWN ROOM

Six months is a good age for a baby to move out of your bedroom and into his or her own space. Your baby is now more likely to wake up when you go to bed or if you turn over in the night. But if you don't have a lot of space, are still breastfeeding or feel that your baby benefits from sleeping near you, you may prefer to go on sharing a room for longer.

Avoid changing your baby's sleeping arrangements when in the throes of separation anxiety, during teething

or illness, or if the baby is experiencing change of another kind – for example, a new carer – and make sure that the baby is happy in the new room before you move the cot there. Buy or borrow a few new toys and place some favourite books there to make it fun. Spend as much time as possible in the room during the day for at least a week before moving the baby in. If your baby is easy to settle, you can use the new bedroom for daytime naps – in the buggy or a travel cot if you have one.

Move the cot in the morning. Put a couple of interesting activity toys in it plus one or two old favourites, including your baby's comforter if he or she has one. Give the baby two or three play sessions in the cot during the day. Stay nearby for these; if possible, busy yourself in the room so that the baby plays independently. Take the baby out as soon as he or she starts to get fed up. Follow your usual bedtime routine, and then put your baby to bed at the usual time in the cot. If he or she wakes up, make sure you get there quickly to help him or her settle back to sleep. You could consider putting a spare bed or mattress in the baby's room, so that you can sleep there if the baby becomes distressed rather than taking him or her back to your room.

Don't forget to give your baby plenty of attention and cuddles during the day to help him or her feel secure. Avoid any unusual absences or making any other changes to your baby's routine for a few weeks.

Left: If your baby whimpers in the night, don't pick him or her up too quickly: make sure that the baby really is awake. Try to settle the baby without picking him or her up if you can.

Right: A quiet cuddle before bedtime will help to get your baby into a relaxed state conducive to sleep. Make this the final thing you do, after toothbrushing or a nappy change.

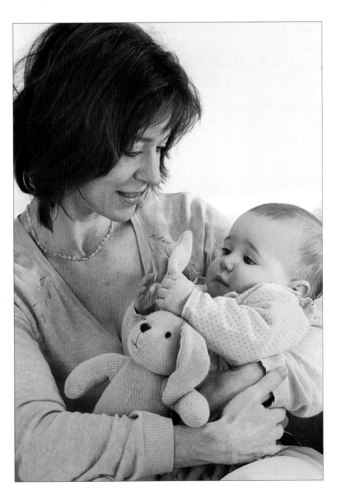

Improving sleep in an older baby

How you deal with broken nights depends very much on whether you think a baby should learn to fit in with your routine or feel that it is your job as a parent to tend to the baby's needs, even when it causes you a lot of inconvenience. Both attitudes have their supporters, but whatever you do, some sleepless nights are inevitable. Here are some simple ways to minimize them.

The baby may be getting hungry. Try to ensure that he or she gets enough food during the day by prioritizing mealtimes and by giving a full breastfeed or a bottle at bedtime. If the baby falls asleep during this feed, give it a little earlier – before a bath or story.

Check that your baby's bedroom is conducive to sleep. Some babies are more sensitive than others and need a carefully controlled environment in order to get through the night. Is it dark and warm enough? If your baby pulls the covers off and then wakes up because it is cold,

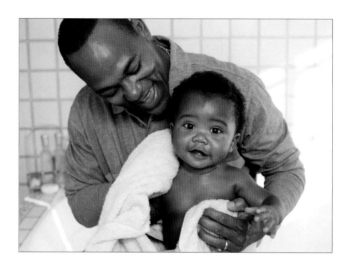

A warm bath is the ideal way for many babies to wind down before bedtime. You can encourage sleepiness by adding a couple of drops of lavender or chamomile essential oils, well diluted in a carrier oil or in milk.

consider using a baby sleeping bag instead of blankets. Your baby may need quiet to sleep, but some find it easier to drop off if there is some noise – try leaving the door open so that the baby can hear the household sounds, or leave a ticking clock, a soothing musical mobile or a radio turned down low. A nightlight can also help some babies to sleep better.

Have a consistent bedtime routine that allows your baby to wind down properly – say, a warm bath, a story or song on your lap and then a feed. If you can, get your baby into bed while sleepy but still awake, to learn to drop off on his or her own (this is hard if you are breastfeeding and have a baby who falls asleep at the breast). Introduce a comforter if your baby doesn't already use one. This can be particularly useful if you are trying to move your baby into a cot from your family bed. And if you are breastfeeding and want to stop night feeds, get your partner or a supportive helper to attend to the baby during the night for a while.

LIGHT MORNINGS

Early-morning waking is very common, especially in summer, and it is hard to handle. Generally speaking it doesn't work to start putting your baby to bed later – he or she will almost certainly wake up at the same time. The most helpful thing that you can do is to ensure your baby's room is really dark – put up blackout blinds or curtain lining to eliminate the first chinks of light. It is also a good idea to treat all feeds before, say, 6 am as quiet night feeds. You can also try putting a couple of toys in the baby's cot so that he or she discovers them on awakening. You may find that he or she will then play happily in the cot for 20 minutes or so while you enjoy a few precious minutes' extra sleep.

ADOPTING A COMFORTER

You can encourage your baby to adopt a comforter if you think it will make settling at night easier. Over time your baby will associate it with love and sleep, but remember that once this association is made, the comforter will be extremely important to your child – you won't be able to go away for a night without it.

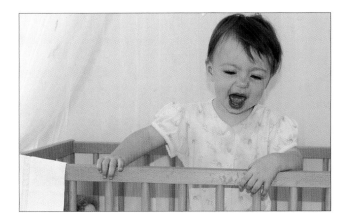

Children do tend to wake up earlier than their parents, and protest vigorously if they don't get a response.

Make sure that you are allowing your baby the opportunity to settle him or herself. It's easy to get into the habit of picking up your baby as soon as he or she makes a sound, especially if the baby is sharing your room. But babies often whimper, cry out or cough in their sleep without actually waking up properly. Wait for a few moments and listen – your baby may continue sleeping if you do not disturb him or her unnecessarily.

CHECKLIST: WHY IS MY BABY WAKING UP?
Here are some of the reasons why an unbroken night's sleep might be eluding you and your baby.
Hunger. If your baby wakes up and won't settle, he or she may need a feed. Keep the room dark as you feed and put the baby back to bed straight away.
Comfort feeding. Lots of breastfed babies wake up several times a night to nurse. Sometimes this is hunger but it can also be because they enjoy having their relaxed mother to themselves.
Anxiety. Babies may become more restless if they are unsettled by a major change – starting at nursery, for example. If your baby is experiencing separation anxiety, he or she may start to resist going to bed.
Developmental leaps. Your baby may be more wakeful at night when acquiring a new skill.
External disturbances. An older baby may be disturbed by noises or by your movements. This doesn't mean your home has to be kept silent – normal household noises can be comforting.
Physical needs. Teething pain – and any accompanying fever – can make for very disturbed nights. Your baby may also wake if too hot or cold, with a soiled or very full nappy, or if he or she is ill. If you think your baby's wakefulness may be due to illness, see your doctor.
Habit. Babies who are used to being nursed to sleep, for example, may find it hard to drop off on their own when they wake up at night.

A responsible older sibling may be willing to amuse the baby for a short period so that you can get more sleep.

If your baby doesn't seem to like being in the cot, let him or her have a few play sessions there during the day while you potter about in the room. However, take most of the toys out of the cot at bedtime: one stuffed animal or a comforter is enough.

Sleep training

All babies wake up from time to time throughout the night. But if your baby is used to being fed or stroked to sleep at bedtime, he or she will need the same help to drop off during the night. The point of sleep training is to teach a baby to get back to sleep on his or her own.

If your baby is continuing to wake up several times a night, you may decide that now is the time to take action. Unless there is a medical reason for the crying – and it is important to check this with your doctor before embarking on sleep training – you should be able to teach your baby to sleep better using one of the methods described below. Set aside at least a week to do it, and don't choose a time when any major change is going on in your child's life, when your partner will be away or you will be going out in the evening.

Don't forget that your baby's sleep, or lack of it, is only really a problem if it is affecting his or her mood and ability to function, or making daily life difficult for you. If you are both happy, it doesn't matter if your child continues to wake up at night – some mothers are happy to give night feeds for the first year and beyond.

If you can, continue with the method throughout the night. But it is also fine to do the sleep plan until a certain time – 1 am, say – and then to revert to your usual methods if you find that easier. Stick with your sleep plan for at least a week if you can, to instil the idea that once your baby goes into the cot, he or she stays there. It is important that you and your partner agree your approach to sleep training if you are both going to be involved.

Sleep training aims to teach a baby to get to sleep without your help, so that he or she doesn't need to disturb you during the night unless something is wrong.

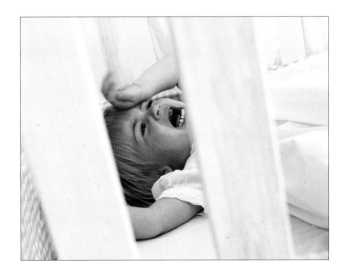

Make a decision about what you want, and work out what steps you are going to take to get there. Be clear about who is going to do what – it is difficult to make sensible decisions when you are faced with a crying child at 3am.

CONTROLLED CRYING

This is the sleep-training method recommended by many health professionals. It doesn't involve leaving your baby to scream unattended for a long time; instead you keep checking so that your baby knows you are there. This can make the baby furious – if you are coming in, why aren't you picking him or her up? – and the process can take longer than if you simply leave the child to scream it out. But it won't leave your baby feeling abandoned and it will mean you can check that nothing else is wrong – such as wind, or a lost dummy (pacifier) or comforter.

Controlled crying is stressful for everyone concerned, so try gentler methods first. If you do decide to do it, be certain that it is the right choice for both parent(s) and child. Be clear with your partner about who is going to do what before you begin. Stick to the method for at least four days – crying often peaks on the third. Remember that you can adapt the method to suit yourself. For example, you may decide that ten minutes is your limit for crying or that you will stroke your baby when you go in.

1 Follow a bedtime routine and put the baby to bed when sleepy and relaxed. Kiss goodnight and leave the room.

2 If the baby cries, wait one minute then return. You can shush, but don't linger or pick up. Gradually increase the time that you leave the baby to cry – to two minutes, then three, then five, then eight, ten and finally 15. Don't leave the baby crying any longer than 15 minutes at a time.

3 Be resolute – if you give in, your baby will hold out for longer the next time you try the method. Continue checking every 15 minutes until your baby falls asleep.

4 If your baby wakes up later in the night, go through the same process of checking and leaving for increasing periods of time, up to 15 minutes. Never just leave your baby crying without checking.

> **CAUTION**
> Any form of sleep training is stressful. Be clear about what you want to achieve and stay calm. It works best if one person tackles each night, but it is a good idea to have your partner or a supportive helper on hand to take over if you become overwhelmed.

Settling a reluctant baby

Some babies do not want to go to bed on their own because it means being away from you. They may be in the habit of falling asleep while breastfeeding, or coming into bed with you to get to sleep. Unless you want to sleep with your baby and go to bed very early every night, this is something you do need to tackle. Here is a gentle way to settle a reluctant baby. It involves gradually reducing the amount of soothing you do. Once you are down to the bare minimum, you should find that your baby finds it easier to drop off on his or her own.

1 Go through your usual bedtime routine. Cuddle or feed until your baby is sleepy, and then put him or her in the cot. Stay in contact – leave one hand underneath the baby's back and stroke his or her head or tummy with the other. Soothe the baby verbally at the same time – try shushing, repeating a key phrase such as "Sleepy time", or singing the same song.

2 If your baby gets very distressed, you may want to pick him or her up. Once comforted, put the baby back in the cot straight away – you may have to do this many times before he or she becomes calmer. If your baby is standing up, lie him or her down. Often a baby will scramble up again immediately. Just keep lying them down again until he or she gets the message and gives in.

3 Once your baby is lying down, keep reassuring them. Combine physical comfort with verbal soothing, reducing the volume as your baby calms down. Stay calm yourself – do some deep breathing if you need to. You should find that the baby's protests gradually become less vocal and insistent, but it can take a lot of patient perseverance before this happens.

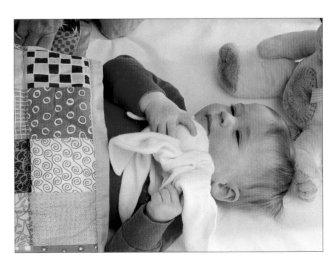

4 Once the baby is calm and sleepy, try stroking your hand from the forehead downwards. As your hand passes over the baby's eyes, they automatically shut and this can help lull him or her into sleep. Continue the verbal soothing, becoming quieter and quieter as the baby drifts off. Slowly remove your hand as you continue to shush or sing. Stand by the cot for a few minutes before retreating.

5 After a few days, your baby should be quietened more easily. Once he or she starts to go into the cot calmly, try simply sitting beside the cot and comforting him or her from a distance – but still go and offer physical comfort if he or she cries. Eventually, when you judge the time is right, you may be able to leave the room and let the baby drift off alone.

Development and play

> 66 This new ability to get around will make your baby more physically independent, but emotionally his or her attachment to you will grow. 99

The second half-year of your baby's life is a most eventful time. In the space of a few short months he or she will learn to sit up, and then to get about – by crawling, bottom-shuffling or simply wriggling across the floor. No longer does your baby have to wait to be moved or given interesting things to examine – now he or she can just go and get them.

At some point during these months, your baby will discover how to pull up to a standing position, and will figure out how to edge around a room by holding on to the furniture. This new ability to get around will make your baby more physically independent, but emotionally his or her attachment to you will grow, and a strong bond will also develop with other important people in the baby's life.

Excitingly, your baby will also have some new ways to interact with you. Older babies understand the word "no", although they may not always obey it, and they know their own names and turn round when you call them. By the end of the first year, many

Cruising gives your baby a degree of independence, which he or she will exercise to the full. Standing and moving about will become a favourite activity.

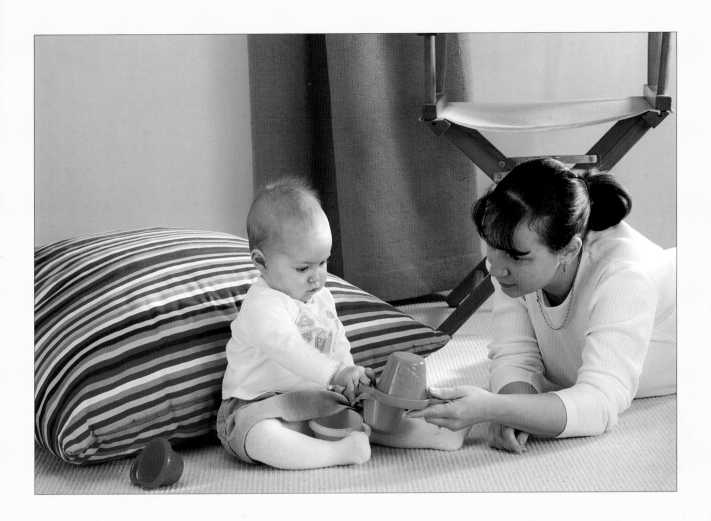

babies can use a few hand signals to communicate: they may wave goodbye, point at something they want and clap hands. Most babies love showing off these new skills, especially when they meet with approval and delight in those around them.

All these new developments mean that outings become more fun. Your increasingly curious and sociable baby will really enjoy music classes now he or she can see what is going on, and will love to shake a percussion instrument or clap with the music. Baby gyms provide your baby with the opportunity for a bit of rough and tumble.

At a developmental review (well-child visit), during this time you will be asked about your baby's eating and sleeping and new achievements. This is a good opportunity to raise any concerns you may have.

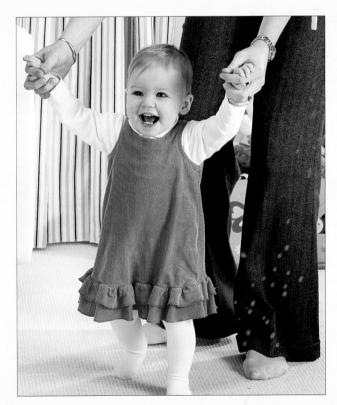

Top: The time when your baby sits up but cannot yet move about is probably the easiest stage of parenthood. He or she will be contented to sit and explore toys.

Babies who are beginning to stand will love being walked round. Some babies start walking independently, though most won't do this until well after one year.

Sitting and crawling

Babies love to sit, but it usually takes six months before they can stay upright by themselves. Before then, you can help your baby practise by sitting him or her in a circle of cushions or rolled-up blankets; the baby will rock from side to side as he or she tries to balance.

Sitting is great fun for babies because it gives a much more comprehensive view of what is going on. It also allows them to stretch further to grab interesting objects, and of course their hands are now free for exploring any item within reach. Expect your sitting baby to topple over a lot. Even after mastering the skill, it takes time to learn exactly how far he or she can reach out without tipping over. Until then, continue to use cushions or rolled-up blankets to give a soft landing. Stay close by: if your baby falls head-down into a pile of cushions in an awkward position, he or she could get stuck.

Most babies are at least nine months old before they can move from a lying-down position to sitting up, without help. Before this they will use any means available to haul themselves up, whether this is your hands, a tablecloth or the sides of a buggy. Be vigilant about strapping your baby into the buggy and highchair, so that he or she can't fall out. If you are still sitting your baby on a sofa or bed, it is definitely time to stop: he or she could easily tip on to the floor.

Babies who are just learning to sit haven't yet worked out how far they can lean forwards without falling over. They need a helping hand to explore safely.

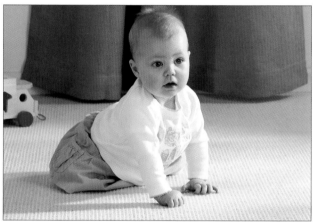

Because motor control develops from the head down, babies' arms are much stronger than their legs at first. So they may use their arms to pull themselves along, commando-style, before they start to crawl properly.

CRAWLING

Not all babies crawl. Some get about by shuffling on their bottoms, using one hand to push themselves forward. Others travel on their hands and feet with their bottoms

---

CHECKLIST: SAFETY FOR MOBILE BABIES
- Dress your baby in clothes that cover the knees to protect them from hard surfaces or carpet.
- Check wooden floors for splinters, gaps and any protruding nails.
- Put up stair gates.
- Check your child proofing.
- Remember that babies can learn a new skill quite suddenly. If your baby is getting ready to crawl, take precautions straight away

MOBILITY

Babies vary so much in when and how they start to get mobile that crawling isn't included as one of the developmental milestones. It doesn't matter if your baby doesn't crawl, just so long as he or she finds some way of moving around. But if your baby isn't mobile by the age of one, or doesn't seem to use all his or her arms and legs when moving, you should consult a health professional. Remember that premature babies often do things later than other babies born at the same time.

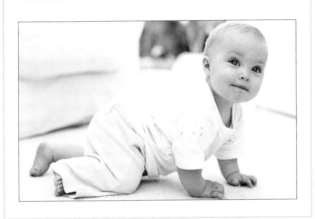

high in the air – the "bear-walk". And some cut out this middle stage altogether, going straight from sitting to cruising and walking. Babies who do crawl usually start between eight and ten months, but they start to practise well before this. Often they start by pushing themselves up on their hands and knees when they are lying on their stomachs. It can take them many weeks to figure out how to move forwards from this position: they tend to rock backwards and forwards without going anywhere.

When they do start to move, it is often backwards. This is because their arms are stronger than their legs, but they soon learn how to push with their knees to move forwards. And once they work out how to use opposite arms and legs together, they can go much faster.

You can't help a baby to crawl, but you can provide the opportunities to practise and a safe space to play in, and put the baby down on his or her front often. Placing an interesting toy just out of reach can encourage a baby to try to move forwards. Once crawling starts, it is fun to make a mini obstacle course using cushions, which your baby then has to go around or climb over in order to get to you or to a favourite toy. This can help build confidence and improve balance and coordination, but do help out if your baby gets stuck or frustrated.

CHILDPROOFING YOUR HOME

It is a good idea to crawl around your living spaces to look for hazards such as trailing cords, sharp corners and uncovered plug sockets. A mobile baby will investigate

Once your baby becomes mobile, you will need to make sure that your home is safe and be on the lookout for hazards when you are out. Keep one step ahead of your baby's development, since he or she may progress quite suddenly.

anything on the floor, so check for dropped coins and stray objects under sofas and so on. Put up stair gates, but once your baby is confidently mobile, let him or her practise crawling up stairs while you follow. You can also let your baby come down the stairs feet-first on his or her tummy, so long as you are there in case of a fall. Consider investing in a playpen or travel cot so that you can keep your baby safe if you need to cook, say, when he or she is awake. But don't use it for long periods.

You can buy childproofing safety packs from DIY stores and pharmacies. They include plug guards to prevent your baby poking things in a socket, and corner protectors to cover sharp corners of coffee tables.

Loop up trailing wires of appliances and secure with an elastic band.

Fit catches to cupboard doors so that your toddler can't open them.

Cushions fitted to doors will stop them slamming on little fingers.

Unused electrical sockets can be made safe with these plugs.

The corners of eye-level tables can be cushioned with covers.

Standing and cruising

Babies long to stand on their own two feet in every sense. Moving independently is a great step towards other kinds of independence: they can entertain themselves, reach toys, and set off to find the people that have moved out of view. Babies seem to sense these possibilities for extending their experience: you need only look at the delight on a child's face after negotiating the route from sofa to table leg, from table leg to chair to see this. But learning to walk, like learning to sit, doesn't happen suddenly, it will develop in stages.

From the time they are a few months old, babies love to stand when being held on a lap. They quickly discover that they can bounce up and down if they bend and straighten their knees, and this will probably be one of their first games. At about seven months, they may start to alternate their feet as if they were walking. But most babies haven't yet developed the strength to take their own weight, and they feel insecure if they are "walked" along the ground before they are ready.

Early walkers may take their first steps at eight or nine months, but most babies don't walk unassisted until they are between 12 and 15 months old. A few are older than 18 months when they start.

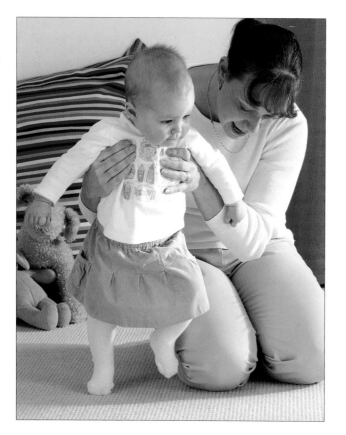

Once your baby starts to cruise, you will probably be astonished by some of the clever ways he or she finds to navigate a room. He or she will use this new skill whenever and wherever possible, so look out for unsafe items on furniture that they will be able to reach.

Most babies have developed enough strength in their legs to stand properly by the time they are about eight or nine months old. But apart from a few early developers, they can't usually maintain the necessary balance to stand independently or to walk. However, they quickly learn to pull themselves up with the help of a chair or the bars of their cots and playpens. They will also enjoy "walking" with your help.

This is a tricky stage for both parent and baby – your baby will repeatedly pull himself or herself up and stand holding on to something at every opportunity. However, the baby hasn't yet worked out how to sit down again. So he or she will shout for you to help – and then promptly stand up again – or will fall on his or her bottom and be shocked by the impact. Be patient: it will take only a few weeks for the baby to figure out how to get back down to the safety of the floor.

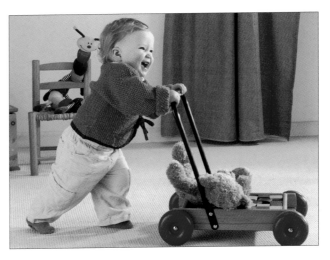

Babies start pulling themselves up from about eight months. But they won't work out how to get down for another month or two.

A toddle truck is the perfect toy for a cruising baby. Look for one that has a stable base and won't tip over. Wooden trucks are often sturdier than plastic ones.

CRUISING

Once your baby can pull up, he or she will soon start to "cruise" – that is, walk while holding on to something. Cruising is likely to become your baby's favourite activity, and he or she will spend many happy minutes walking from one end of the cot to the other, or shuffling along the edge of the sofa.

As he or she gains in confidence, your baby may surprise you with ingenious ways of getting around a room: leaning with the flat of a hand on a wall, stretching up to grab the edge of a table or even pushing a chair along like a walking aid. The baby may navigate to the corner of the refrigerator, say, and then pause to consider how to get to the next piece of furniture. He or she will eventually take the odd unsupported step – like a leap into the unknown – without being aware of it. Your baby is ready to walk, but doesn't quite know it yet.

Don't get shoes until your baby is walking (and even then put them on only when he or she is outside). It is

It's best for babies to learn to walk in bare feet, since this helps with balance and coordination. So hold off putting your baby in shoes indoors.

much better for babies to learn to walk barefoot, which allows them to feel the ground and make the tiny adjustments they need to balance. If socks are necessary to keep a baby's feet warm, make sure they are the right size and the non-slip variety.

STANDING AND CRUISING SAFELY

You can't help a baby to stand or cruise; all you can do is provide a safe environment in which to practise. When ready, your baby will pull himself or herself up by any means possible: it is up to you to ensure it is a safe one.

Move flimsy pieces of furniture out of your living space or put them somewhere out of reach. Your baby can easily pull a light table over, which will not only hurt but will damage his or her confidence.

Remember that once your baby can stand up, he or she will be able to reach for things overhead. So, don't put coffee cups or anything else that can be pulled over on the edge of a table, and take any breakables off low shelves. Abolish tablecloths.

If you haven't been using a baby sleeping bag, don't start now. If your baby isn't used to one, he or she will try to stand up in it and fall over.

CAUTION
Never put your baby in a baby walker. These toys are dangerous: in 1991, almost 28,000 American children were admitted to hospital following accidents with baby walkers. They are not even a good development aid because they tend to reduce a baby's interest in getting around under his or her own steam. They may also even affect the proper development of the leg muscles if used a lot. Reputable baby stores no longer sell them.

Dexterity, doing and thinking

By the age of six months, babies have already learned to grasp an object, put it in the mouth and to pass it from hand to hand. Now, although they still like to put objects in their mouths, they start to use their hands more: watch your baby stroke and pat an object before picking it up, and then shake, roll or bang it on the ground. Try laying your baby on different surfaces – grass, rough carpet, a soft rug, a silky cushion – so he or she can explore the feel. Offer textured books – the baby will quickly work out which part of the page to stroke – as well as toys with interesting textures and shapes.

Over the next few months, your baby's dexterity will improve dramatically. Babies learn to hold objects in their palms by wrapping their fingers and thumb around them, the thumb working like an extra finger rather than a separate unit. This clumsy hold doesn't allow them to manipulate the object very well. At about seven months, they learn to use the four fingers and the thumb as different units, making it much easier for them to pick up and handle things.

The next stage is to control individual fingers. The first sign that your baby can do this is when he or she starts to point, at about eight months. Some time around nine months, babies learn how to hold an item between index finger and thumb, using the pincer grip that is unique to

Young babies predominantly use their mouths to explore things. But as they become more dextrous, they start to use their hands a lot more.

humans. This enables them to pick up even very tiny objects and to perform sophisticated movements such as turning the pages of a book. You can help your baby to practise the pincer grip by putting a few cooked peas or grains of rice on the highchair's feeding tray at mealtimes: he or she will enjoy the task of picking them up one by

OBJECT PERMANENCE
Very young babies are unaware that anything they cannot see continues to exist. So if they have dropped a toy, say, they won't look for it because in their mind it is no more. Experts differ on when babies start to understand that objects are permanent, but most put it between four and seven months. At some point around this age you will notice that your baby will pull a cloth aside to find a toy that is partially visible. By nine months, a baby will look for a toy even if it is completely hidden. This leap in understanding means that an older baby will be much harder to distract when you take something away. You can help your baby to learn about object permanence by playing variations of the game "peek-a-boo". Cover your face with your hands and then reappear. Hide a squeaky toy under a cloth and make it sound before the baby can see it. Your baby will also enjoy surprising you by playing peek-a-boo back – covering his or her face and then slowly uncovering it. He or she will love it if you respond with surprise.

The pincer movement shows that your baby has control over individual digits. A key sign that it is about to happen is when he or she starts to point.

one. Unfortunately this also goes for any other small item, which will also go in the mouth. This means that you have to be vigilant about what is on the floor: a dropped button or pin could be a real danger.

Your baby will be able to hold only one thing at a time at first and will hold on until he or she loses interest and drops it without noticing. If you try to offer a second toy, he or she will automatically drop the first one in reaching for it. But by seven or eight months, a baby is able to hold two things at once, one in each hand.

Your baby will love to hand things to you. Say "thank you" when he or she puts a toy into your hand – this is the very start of learning to share.

DROPPING AND THROWING

Babies have to learn how to let go of things. At first, they simply hold on until you take an object from them, or they drop it accidentally when their attention is caught by something else. But at about the same time as they learn the pincer grip, they discover how to open their fingers and deliberately drop something that they are holding. This quickly becomes a fun activity they will want to practise again and again. Your baby will love it if you give him or her a small toy and then ask for it back – put your hand under it so you can catch it as it drops.

Be prepared for a few weeks of picking things up whenever your baby is in the highchair – it will add to the baby's fun if you exclaim in mock protest every time you have to do this. You could put a metal tray on the floor where the objects fall so that your baby can hear that different items make different sounds when they hit it: try a metal spoon, a soft toy, a wet flannel and a bouncy ball. To stop your baby's new game becoming a real annoyance, restrict toys for the buggy to those that can be attached to it: the baby can then enjoy throwing them over the side and hauling them back in.

Your baby will also enjoy batting a ball back to you after you throw it. This is a good way to practise hand eye coordination. At first he or she will swipe at the ball and probably miss, but will quickly learn to how to hit it back in your direction.

Once your baby has discovered how to drop things, he or she will enjoy your reaction as they repeatedly hurl toys or dishes down from the high chair.

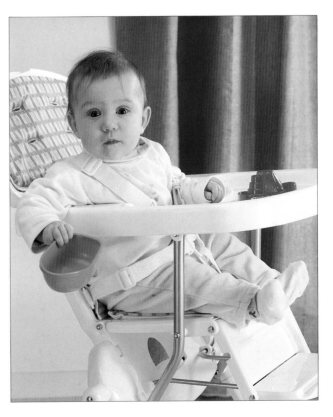

Sociability and language

Now that your baby can sit up and look around, he or she will get a lot more from going out and meeting people. You'll notice that your child starts to become more interested in other babies and children, and may stretch out to touch another baby's hand or face.

Babies love to socialize, and from the age of six months it is important to give them plenty of opportunities to interact with others. This can be as simple as taking your baby with you to the supermarket – it is good to experience positive interactions with strangers, who may smile and play little games while you are in the checkout queue. Your baby will also enjoy classes and parent-and-baby groups, as well as visits to the park to see other children playing.

As the first birthday approaches, you'll notice that your baby becomes more aware of the distinction between familiar people and strangers. For a while, new acquaintances will be scary. One moment the baby may be happy to be cuddled by another adult or to play in front of another baby; the next he or she may be crying for you. This is an aspect of separation anxiety and a normal stage of baby development. Your baby's budding

Your baby won't yet have any understanding of social skills, but you can certainly introduce the concept of being gentle when touching you or another baby. This is the root of empathy, the important notion that you should treat other people kindly.

LANGUAGE SKILLS AT 12 MONTHS
A few babies say their first word by 12 months, but most take longer. Your baby is likely to recognize the following words at one year old.
- His or her own name – the baby may turn towards you when you call it.
- "Hello" and "bye bye" – the baby may start to wave on hearing them.
- "No" – though babies take real delight in ignoring it.
- A few naming words for familiar items – such as "ball", "duck" and "teddy".
- Some basic commands, such as "Give it to mummy."
- Simple questions such as "Where is your nose?" – which the baby may then point to.

awareness of whom he or she belongs to and who belongs to him or her is the beginning of a sense of community, of being part of a family, a friendship group, a nation and a wider world.

LANGUAGE AND THE OLDER BABY
Most babies have started to manifest the rudiments of language by the end of their first year. At this time, you will probably find that your baby babbles more often and in a conversational tone that sounds like real language, as if

Pointing out things of interest and telling your baby about them is something that most parents do instinctively.

One of the first words that babies learn to recognize is their own name. If they hear it often, they will quickly learn that this particular sound means them.

Talking to your child about things that are in front of him of her is the best way to encourage him or her to learn useful everyday words such as "cup".

telling a little story. He or she may even say a few words, though these are unlikely to be perfectly enunciated – for example, "duh" for "duck" or "ook" for "look".

We tend to judge language development by when a baby says the first word, but your child's understanding is racing ahead of his or her ability to articulate. A one-year-old knows a lot more than he or she says, and when a baby chooses to speak the first word is not an indicator of developmental level.

Before your baby speaks, you will see the first green shoots of verbal communication in his or her behaviour. You may notice that the baby listens with greater attention when you talk, and seems to understand words that crop up often. He or she seems to know when you are asking a question – a quizzical expression shows this. And your baby may even know the answer to some frequently asked questions – pointing to a photograph when you say "Where's granny?"; shaking his or her head when you offer another piece of banana (though sometimes this will be for fun, and the baby will take the banana from your hand straight afterwards).

Your baby will also begin to associate certain words with particular situations, which is a stepping-stone towards linking a fixed sound with a definite concept. The baby may, for example, routinely say "Peep-oh" when playing the hiding game or invent words that seem to bear no relation to his or her native language. All this is thrilling for you as a parent. The time when your little baby can tell you what is on his or her mind is just around the corner. Some fascinating and sometimes hilarious conversations lie ahead.

HELPING YOUR BABY TO TALK

Your baby will pick up the meaning of words naturally, but here are some ways you can help.

Talk about things your baby can see. At dinner time, talk about the baby's food, cup, spoon; if you are in the

park, talk about the swings, the children and so on.

Use simple sentences that include key labelling words such as "Here is your teddy", "Pass the teddy to daddy", "Where is teddy?" Your baby has to hear a word in context many times to understand what it signifies.

Get down to your baby's level. Make eye contact when you speak, use big hand gestures, exaggerated facial expressions and a sing-song tone to help your baby grasp the gist of what you are saying.

Spend time talking to your baby each day. Find some time when there are no other distractions (such as older children wanting your attention) or background noise (such as the TV or radio).

Be on the lookout for first words and respond to them, even if they are made up. Your baby will be delighted to see that you know what he or she means.

Second children may spend less one to one time with their parents, but they will benefit from having a sibling to talk to, play with and learn from.

Fun for older babies

New manual dexterity means that your baby can explore toys more thoroughly, and you'll notice that he or she starts to have more interest in what they can do. So the baby may push a toy car along the ground, but place one building brick on top of another.

The best way to encourage your child's learning is to tailor play to abilities. Babies tend to be most interested in skills that they are just about to master or have recently learned. It is up to you to provide activities that are just hard enough to be fun and stimulating: if they are too easy or familiar, the baby will get bored; if they are too difficult, he or she may become upset. You will have to be the judge of when your baby is ready to give them a go.

ROLLING TOYS

A mobile baby will love to chase after toys that roll: a wheeled car or truck, a soft, slow-moving ball or even a toilet roll. Make sure that any rolling toys are too large to fit in the baby's mouth and that they are suitable for this age (don't let your baby play with an older child's car, say, which may have lots of small parts). The baby will also like pulling or pushing toys.

Babies are equally interested in "boy" and "girl" toys, so don't try to limit them. Your little girl may enjoy playing with planes or cars, which she can push along the floor; a little boy may love cuddling a baby doll, which, after all, looks just like him.

In the hands of a baby, a couple of saucepans and a wooden spoon can be magically transformed into a drum kit.

Babies love to knock down towers of bricks, and will eventually start to try building them up for themselves.

TOYS THAT DO THINGS

As your baby gets more dextrous, he or she will enjoy playing with toys that do something, especially if they offer the thrill of surprise. A truck that takes off when you push a button or a jack-in-the-box that pops up when you turn a dial will be a source of real fascination. Let the baby practise setting the toy off: this will help develop dexterity and strength. Toy telephones (and real ones) that ring or buzz are universally popular.

EMPTYING GAMES

Older babies love to empty things out of containers, drawers, cupboards, bags and boxes. To make a game out of this you can fill a fabric shopping bag or a box with a selection of small objects that the baby can take out one by one. Change some of the items every so often to keep the game interesting. As well as toys, you could include things like a wooden spoon, a baby hairbrush, an old notebook, a set of clean, unwanted keys on a ring, an old purse, a plastic pot or an orange. It is a good idea to let the baby help you put them all back in the right place – showing that "tidying up" can be a fun part of playtime.

DISCOVERING WATER

Water is a source of wonder to all babies: it changes shape, cannot be held and glistens in the light. Your baby will love to play pouring games in the bath. Provide a variety of containers of different sizes, and show how to pour water from one to the other. Natural sponges make great bath toys: fill one up and then show your baby how to squeeze the water out of it.

STACKING TOYS

A set of stacking cups will provide months of amusement. At first your baby will simply enjoy exploring similar objects of different sizes. Then he or she will have endless fun putting one of the small cups inside a larger one. This is one way that he or she starts to work out how things are different, and learn important concepts such as big and small. The baby will love to knock down a tower when you build it, and will want to do it over and over again: it is an early way of showing that he or she can change what is happening, giving an enjoyable sense of power and achievement. Eventually, the baby will have a go at putting one cup on top of another, or threading a set of stacking rings on a pole.

MUSICAL TOYS

Babies love things that make noises. Wooden maracas, a tamourine and various shakers will be popular with babies of this age and older, but you don't have to buy musical toys; you can also make your own. An upturned saucepan make a good drum to bang with a wooden spoon, while a few cotton reels in a well-sealed plastic container make a great shaker.

HELPING YOUR BABY ENJOY PLAY

Keep giving your baby new things to play with: babies need lots of variety and get bored if they play with the same toys all the time. But they don't need lots of expensive playthings – your baby really will be as happy exploring a cereal box and other household items as an expensive toy. Reignite your baby's interest in toys he or she has enjoyed by hiding them away for a while and then letting the baby discover them afresh. Allow your baby to make a mess. Babies scatter toys everywhere, and they

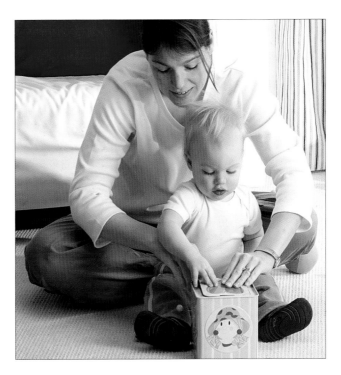

Babies learn by watching other people as well as by exploring things for themselves. So get down on the floor and show your baby how each toy works. He or she may not succeed in copying you, but will have a go – and will remember what to do with that toy next time.

love to empty out a cupboard or a bag of shopping. Be prepared for a less-than-spotless house for a while; you can always tidy up when the baby has gone to bed.

It will help to contain the mess if you restrict emptying games to a special cupboard filled with non-breakable things that can be flung on the floor. Whenever the baby tries to do the same to other cupboards, gently say "No" and lead him or her back to the special cupboard. If you do this consistently, your child will eventually get the message. Be reasonable about what your baby can and cannot do. Move things that you don't want played with, rather than constantly saying "No" every time the baby goes near them.

Left: Stacking cups or rings will give good value for months as a baby's manual skills develop.

Right: As your baby explores objects by handling, he or she starts to work out how things relate to each other. A baby will become totally absorbed in the task of putting a small beaker into a larger one.

section three

health
and safety

When your baby falls ill, as children are bound to do from time to

time, there are plenty of natural treatments you can turn to that do

not involve using chemically refined medicines. With health, as

with food; what you put into your child's body matters. A good

diet and the start of a healthy attitude to food is one of the

greatest gifts you can give your child. It is something that will

stand him or her in good stead for an entire lifetime, and will be a

source of much pleasure and enjoyment. This chapter offers

sensible advice and natural remedies for common health problems

and for a nutritious healthy start to your baby's first foods.

Immunization and supplements

The subject of immunization causes parents a lot of anxiety, but in a sense there is nothing unnatural about it: what you are doing is introducing a small dose of a disease into the body so that the immune system can develop antibodies to it. This is exactly what the body does when it encounters a disease "accidentally", except that with vaccination the body does not go through the dangers and unpleasantness of illness.

There is no doubt that we all have benefited from a widespread vaccination programme: smallpox has been eradicated worldwide, and diseases such as polio and diphtheria are now largely unknown in developed countries. However, there is much debate about the wisdom of vaccinating very young children. Some natural practitioners say that the standard practice of immunizing babies against several diseases at once overloads their immature immune systems and can lead to an increased risk of problems such as asthma, eczema and allergy later on. And parents worry about the possibility of side effects. Controversy over the MMR jab, which was linked to autism in one British study, caused many parents to decide not to give it to their children. This study has been widely discredited and intensive research has not found a link. Generally speaking, the risk of serious side effects from a vaccine is much smaller than the risk from diseases such as measles.

Every parent has to make an individual decision about what is right for a child. There are four options:

Following the standard vaccination programme. This is what the vast majority of doctors recommend.

Delaying vaccinations. Some people prefer to give vaccinations when the child is older, to give the immune system a chance to strengthen. This may make you feel more comfortable, especially if there is a family history

of allergy or allergy-related illnesses. However, your child will obviously not be protected in the meantime.

Having selected vaccinations. Some parents prefer to avoid giving children all-in-one shots, and choose not to vaccinate against certain diseases. It is worth bearing in mind that single-vaccine injections may not have been tested as rigorously as the standard injections.

Not vaccinating. If you feel strongly that vaccination is not right for your child, then you may decide not to do it

Vaccination jabs are usually given in the thigh. Some children barely notice them; others get upset but can usually be quickly soothed.

Giving children a specially developed multi-vitamin supplement will ensure that they receive the right amount of vitamins and minerals in their diet.

THE IMMUNIZATION PROGRAMME (UK)

2 months	One shot for diphtheria, tetanus, pertussis (whooping cough), haemophilus influenza B (HIB), polio
	One shot for meningitis C
3 months	One shot for diphtheria, tetanus, pertussis, HIB
	One shot for meningitis C
4 months	One shot for diphtheria, tetanus, pertussis, HIB, polio
	One shot for meningitis C
13 months	Measles, mumps and rubella (MMR)
3–5 years	One shot for diphtheria, tetanus, pertussis, HIB
	One shot for MMR

THE IMMUNIZATION PROGRAMME (US)

Birth–2 months	Hepatitis B (1/3)
2 months	Diphtheria, tetanus, pertussis (1/5)
	HIB (1/4)
	Polio (1/4)
	Hepatitis B (2/3)
	Pneumococcal conjugate (PCV7) (1/4)
4 months	Diphtheria, tetanus, pertussis (2/5)
	HIB (2/4)
	Polio (2/4)
	PCV7 (2/4)
6 months	Diphtheria, tetanus, pertussis (3/5)
	HIB (3/4)
	PCV7 (3/4)
12 months	Hepatitis B (3/3)
	Varicella (chickenpox)
	MMR (1/2)
6–23 months	Influenza (annual shot)
15–18 months	HIB (4/4)
	Polio (3/4)
	PCV7 (4/4)
	Diphtheria, tetanus, pertussis (4/5)
2 years +	Hepatitis A, for specific groups only (1/2)
2 1/2 years +	Hepatitis A, for specific groups only (2/2)
2–5 years	Pneumococcal polysaccaride (PPV23), high risk only (1/2)
4–6 years	Diphtheria, tetanus, pertussis (5/5)
	Polio (4/4)
	MMR (2/2)

at all. Ensuring your child is as healthy as possible is vital: a child with a robust immune system is likely to react to infection less severely. Seek advice from a naturopath, nutritional therapist or homeopath on ways to help support your child's immune system.

NUTRITIONAL SUPPLEMENTS FOR CHILDREN

Many nutritionists maintain that you can get all the nutrients you need from a good mixed diet. However, the mineral and vitamin content of fresh produce has dropped in recent years as the soil in which food is grown has become depleted. Giving children a daily multimineral, multivitamin supplement helps to ensure that they get enough health-giving trace elements, such as zinc.

Minerals work in combination inside the body, so it is not a good idea to give single-mineral supplements without professional advice: giving a dose of one mineral could lead to a deficiency in another. Giving high doses of certain vitamins can also be dangerous. If you think that your child needs a particular nutrient, it is best to seek advice from a qualified nutritional therapist or your doctor.

Probiotics work to replenish levels of good bacteria in the gut, which help with digestion. They can be very useful if your child has had a stomach upset or been on antibiotics. Fish oils (omega-3), or a vegetarian equivalent such as flaxseed, can be beneficial if your child will not eat oily fish. A deficiency in omega-3 oils may contribute to behavioural problems (including hyperactivity) and conditions such as eczema and asthma.

A liquid vitamin formulation, which is gentle on the stomach and suitable for children, can be bought from health food stores; babies can be given vitamin drops.

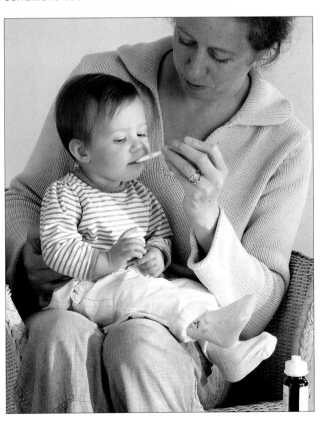

Natural medication

There's no doubt that modern medicine can be useful when your child is very ill. But it is wise to refrain from giving medication when it is not strictly necessary. Some medicines – such as cough mixtures – interrupt the workings of the immune system. Others, such as antibiotics, tend to be overused to the extent that they can be rendered impotent.

Natural remedies and common-sense measures can be just as good as conventional medicines in soothing certain symptoms and encouraging healing. And complementary therapies can encourage the body's natural ability to mend itself. Parents often feel more comfortable using natural methods to treat their children because they tend to have a gentler action than conventional medicines. But it is essential to take a balanced view. For example, not all natural remedies are gentle: some are toxic if taken in large quantities or are not advisable for babies or young children. And if your child is seriously ill, natural remedies are unlikely to help and urgent medical attention should always be sought.

GIVING MEDICATION

Doctors have different attitudes towards natural remedies and complementary therapies. If possible, find a doctor who is open-minded and try to build a good and respectful relationship so that you can discuss alternative methods. If you know that your doctor generally agrees with a cautious approach to medication, you will also feel more confident about taking advice if he or she urges conventional treatment.

Always ask how a medicine works if you are going to give it to your baby. You should know why you are giving it. Ask whether there are any side effects, so you can be on the lookout for them. If your baby is already on medication – or is taking natural remedies – always mention it to the doctor. Check that the medicine is really necessary in your baby's case. Sometimes a doctor may prescribe medication because that is what most parents expect, not because he or she feels it is essential treatment. Ask whether alternative medicines or approaches could work. Your doctor may be happy for you to delay giving antibiotics, say, for 24 hours to see if your child's condition improves on its own.

When you do give medication, don't forget to give every dose on time. Set an alarm to remind you, and keep a record of every dose you give. Don't stop the medication if your baby starts to feel better. Antibiotics, for example, need to be taken for a set number of days in order to kill the bacteria and prevent infection recurring. On the other hand, sometimes the recommended course is longer than strictly necessary, to allow for a margin of error: check with your doctor whether you could stop a course a day or two earlier.

HIGH TEMPERATURE

The conventional response to a temperature is to give paracetamol (acetaminophen) in order to bring it down again. It is worth considering whether this is necessary, and whether simple natural measures may be sufficient. Fever is part of the body's natural response to infection. It helps to increase the number of disease-fighting white blood cells in the bloodstream, and boosts the level of the antiviral substance interferon. Once the immune system has beaten the infection, the body's thermostat will reset itself and your baby's temperature will return to normal.

A child may have a raised temperature simply because he or she has too many clothes on. Taking off a layer or two and opening a window may be all you need to do to combat a slightly raised temperature. Teething and vaccination may also cause a rise in body temperature.

> **CAUTION**
> A very high temperature in a child can cause a fit (febrile convulsion). In the event of a seizure, lay your child on one side and remove anything in his or her mouth. Call an ambulance.

If you need to give a young baby medicine, use a sterilized syringe. Hold it against your baby's bottom lip and depress the plunger slowly so that the medicine doesn't hit the back of the throat hard.

Your child needs a strong immune system in order to cope with all the bugs he or she comes across in daily life. One study found that the more fevers children had in the first year of life, the less likely they were to develop allergies later on. So it may be unwise to give medicines that, in the long term, may interfere with this natural mechanism for dealing with disease.

WHEN TO CALL A DOCTOR
Seek medical advice if a baby under three months has a fever, or if a child has a fever that is over 39°C/102°F, lasts

MANAGING FEVER NATURALLY
A fever can be dangerous if it gets very high and a raised temperature can also be uncomfortable. Follow these steps to help to lower a fever naturally.

1 Remove your child's clothing. Turn down any heating and ventilate the room to cool it.

2 Sponge your child down using tepid water; don't use cold water, as this will cause the blood vessels to contract, and so raise the core temperature of the body. Leave the water to evaporate rather than drying with a towel.

3 Dress your child in minimum clothing and, if he or she is in bed, cover with a sheet or light blanket. Give lots of fluid: frequent breastfeeds or extra drinks of cooled, boiled water for a baby; lots of cool drinks for older children. Encourage your child to sip drinks, as gulping could induce vomiting.

4 Check your child's temperature in half an hour, and then every hour or two.

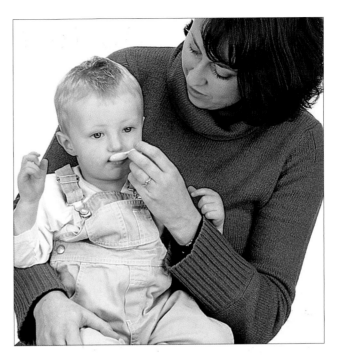

Older babies and children may prefer to take medicine from a spoon rather than syringe; use a proper measuring spoon to be sure of giving the correct dose.

for longer than 24 hours or seems to be steadily increasing. If you do decide to give medication, children's paracetamol (acetaminophen), suitable for babies over two months, is milder than chidren's ibuprofen. Never give a child aspirin, which is linked with the rare and potentially fatal disease Reye's syndrome.

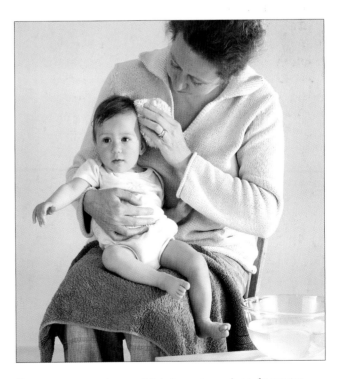

If you are sponging a child down to reduce fever, try adding 2 drops of lavender or chamomile essential oil dissolved in 20ml/4 tsp full-fat milk to the water: these oils reduce fever and encourage sleep.

Natural first aid

All children have tumbles and minor accidents, and you are bound to have to deal with grazed knees, burns and cuts. Natural remedies help speed healing and can also soothe an unhappy child. But don't hesitate to get medical attention if your child has had a bad fall or if you cannot easily treat the injury yourself.

A NATURAL FIRST-AID BOX

These are some of the most useful natural remedies to have to hand.

Aloe vera gel. A herbal remedy for burns and rashes. Aloe vera has natural antiseptic, antibiotic and anti-inflammatory properties. You can also use the fresh sap of an aloe vera leaf.

Arnica. This homeopathic remedy

STANDARD FIRST-AID ITEMS

You can buy a first-aid kit from pharmacists, but it is easy to make your own. Get a rigid, closable box and fill it with the following basic items: scissors, safety pins, tweezers, cotton wool, bandages, absorbent dressings, gauze dressings and assorted plasters.

comes in cream and tablet form, and it is worth getting both. The cream is good for bruises; the tablets are also helpful for bruises as well as sprains, shock after an injury, and nosebleeds.

Calendula cream. A natural antifungal and antiseptic cream that fights infection. Calendula is good for minor skin complaints such as burns, blisters and insect bites and stings.

Chamomilla. A homeopathic remedy for teething pain and sleeplessness. Diluted chamomile tea can also be useful, both to sip and for compresses.

Distilled witch hazel. A widely available liquid herbal remedy that is good for bites, stings, bruises and sprains.

Lavender oil. A multipurpose essential oil that has antibacterial and anti-inflammatory qualities; it is good for sleeplessness, minor skin problems and headaches.

Rescue Remedy. This gentle blend of flower essences is great for calming upset children after an accident. Put four drops in water and give to your child to sip.

Most children enjoy having a "magic" cream smoothed over their hurts. Arnica will help to speed healing from bruising.

Roman chamomile oil. A soothing essential oil that helps with sleeplessness, muscle strain and skin problems.

Tea tree oil. An antibacterial and antifungal essential oil that helps to prevent infection.

Honey has been used for centuries as a natural antiseptic, it also has anti-inflammatory qualities, and is a natural antihistamine.

MAKING A LAVENDER COMPRESS

1 Fill a bowl with very cold water and add a handful of ice cubes.
2 Add a few drops of lavender oil diluted in 15ml/1 tbsp full-fat milk.
3 Dip a clean facecloth into the scented water.
4 Squeeze out excess water and apply to the bruised area. Dip the cloth frequently to keep it cold. Apply for a maximum of 10 minutes in total. Reapply every few hours as necessary.

A few drops of Rescue Remedy added to a cup of water can help soothe minor shocks and upsets.

CUTS AND GRAZES

Most cuts are minor wounds that heal quickly but you should always clean the damaged skin to prevent infection. Grazes often occur when the child has slid along the ground after a fall, so they may contain bits of dirt or grit, which will all need to be removed.

What to do. Fill a small bowl with warm water, add a couple of drops of tea tree oil and use to bathe the wound, or simply wash under running water. Press a folded pad of gauze or similar over the area to stop bleeding (don't use cotton wool (cotton balls) as the fibres may stick). Smooth a little Calendula cream over the cleaned area before covering with a plaster. You can also apply honey: ideally use manuka honey, which has a marked antibacterial and anti-inflammatory action.

When to seek help. Seek medical attention if the cut is very deep, there are objects embedded in it that you cannot easily remove, it doesn't stop bleeding when a dressing is applied or if it covers a large area.

BRUISES

When the blood vessels under the skin are damaged, blood seeps out into the surrounding tissues, causing bruising. Some children bruise more easily than others. Including more fruits and vegetables in the diet can help, since these foods are known to contain vitamin C and bioflavonoids, which help to strengthen the walls of blood vessels.

What to do. Apply a cold lavender compress to the skin for a few minutes to reduce swelling. A packet of frozen peas wrapped in a towel will also work well. Don't hold a compress against your child's skin for longer than 10 minutes. To encourage healing, smooth Arnica cream on the bruise three times a day. You can also give an Arnica tablet immediately after the injury to help with the shock, and every two hours during daytime for the next 48 hours.

When to seek help. See a doctor if you suspect a broken bone, or if the pain is worse 24 hours later. Frequent bruising is occasionally due to a problem with blood clotting: see your doctor if your child bruises very easily and unusually.

NOSEBLEEDS

A nosebleed happens when the delicate blood vessels that line the nose are damaged by a blow, frequent nose-blowing or picking, or inflammation caused by a cold. If your child has nosebleeds often, try giving more fruits and vegetables to increase his or her intake of vitamin C and bioflavonoids.

What to do. Get your child to lean forwards (not backwards), and gently pinch the fleshy part just under the bridge of the nose for 10–15 minutes. Release, repeat if bleeding continues. Arnica tablets can be given after a nosebleed, or daily for frequent bleeds. Rescue Remedy helps soothe any shock.

When to seek help. Take your child to hospital if a nosebleed occurs after a blow to the head, or if the bleeding doesn't stop within half an hour. See a doctor if your child has frequent nosebleeds.

A pack of frozen peas wrapped in a muslin makes a makeshift icepack.

CHOKING

A sudden fit of coughing may mean your child is choking on a piece of food or other small item. The natural instinct to give someone who is choking a slap on the back is a good one, but encourage a child to cough first – this is often enough to remove an obstruction. Check the mouth and remove the obstruction if you can see it: don't feel for it with your fingers – you may damage the throat or push the obstruction in further.

If you do need to slap the child on the back, get him to bend over (or bend him over your knee) and slap between the shoulderblades. If a baby is choking, hold him face-down along your forearm so that the head is facing downwards and use two fingers to tap sharply between the shoulder blades.

All parents worry about choking and it is worth learning how to do chest compressions and life-saving procedures in the very unlikely event that back slaps don't clear the obstruction. You can do a simple first-aid course specifically for babies and children; this usually involves practising the techniques on a life-sized model. Courses are run by voluntary organizations such as St John Ambulance (Red Cross) and are aimed at parents and carers. Often there are child care facilities.

SPRAINS AND STRAINS

A sprain is an injury to the ligaments of a joint, while a strain is an injury to a muscle. It's quite difficult to tell the difference between a strain or sprain and a fracture, especially in young children, whose bones may bend rather than break. If in doubt, seek medical advice.

What to do. Get your child to sit or lie down. Apply a cold lavender or chamomile compress or ice pack for up to 10 minutes. Place a thick wad of cotton wool or other soft pad against the injury and bandage firmly, or put on an elastic bandage to compress. Then elevate the

injured part to reduce swelling. Give Arnica for shock and to encourage healing; Rhus tox is another good homeopathic remedy for sprains and strains. Apply Arnica cream or comfrey ointment over the area (only if the skin is unbroken). Rescue Remedy will help soothe any upset.

Caution. Be sure that you do not bandage so tightly that you cut off the circulation. To check, press on an uninjured area of skin below the bandaged area. If it takes more than three seconds for colour to return, your bandage is probably too tight.

When to seek help. Get medical advice if you suspect a fracture or if the pain doesn't subside at all after the treatment.

WASP AND BEE STINGS

These stings can be very painful.
What to do. If you can see a sting in

Arnica cream and tablets help to speed healing for a strain or sprain.

If you need to bandage a sprain, use a thick wad of gauze or cotton wool to cushion the wound first.

your child's skin, remove it carefully. Put a little iced water in a bowl and add a few drops of lavender or tea tree oil diluted in 15ml/1 tbsp full-fat milk. Dip cotton wool in the water and apply to the area every 10 minutes or so until the pain subsides. Other easily available natural remedies for bee stings include witch hazel, bicarbonate of soda or crushed garlic; wasp stings can be helped by applying witch hazel, cider vinegar or lemon juice. The homeopathic remedy Apis can be given to help with the after-effects of a sting.

When to seek help. If your child is allergic to wasp or bee stings, he or she may go into anaphylactic shock, needing urgent medical attention.

INSECT BITES

Gnat, ant or mosquito bites can be very itchy.
What to do. Witch hazel is a good treatment for insect bites. Rescue Remedy can be applied to the bite. Mosquito bites can be soothed with cider vinegar or lemon juice.
Prevention. Before dusk, when mosquitoes are most active, cover up your child in clothes of closely woven, lightly coloured fabric. You can get eucalyptus-based repellents

Remove a bee sting by scraping it off with a credit card or by pressing your thumb into the neighbouring skin and pushing it sideways. Don't try to pull it out with tweezers: this can squeeze any poison left in the sting into your child's skin. Suck out any poison before treating.

suitable for children from health food stores. Burning citronella oil in a vaporizer or using citronella candles is also helpful.

BURNS

Minor (first-degree) burns affect only the top layer of skin, which reddens but does not blister or swell. They can be treated at home.

What to do. Place the burned area under cold, running water for 10 minutes. Apply aloe vera gel, Calendula cream, or lavender oil

Acidic lemon juice or cider vinegar can take the sting out of a mosquito bite.

You can get witchhazel in the traditional tincture form or in handy tubes of gel.

diluted in full-fat milk to ease pain and speed healing. Give Rescue Remedy or Arnica for the shock.

When to seek help. If the burn is larger than the child's palm or if the pain gets worse after treatment, seek immediate medical advice. If the skin is moist, swollen or blistered, the burn may have reached underlying areas of skin (second-degree burn); if the child feels no pain after a burn but the area is red, white, yellow or darkened, the nerves may be damaged (third-degree burn). Seek urgent medical advice.

SUNBURN

It's important to protect your child's delicate skin from the sun. If it gets too much sunlight, the skin will be red, hot and sore.

What to do. Bathe the skin in cool water to which you have added a couple of drops of lavender oil diluted in full-fat milk. Add a few drops of lavender oil to aloe vera gel and smooth over the affected area. The homeopathic remedy Sol is good for mild sunburn.

When to seek help. Seek immediate medical advice if the skin has blistered, or if your child develops a high temperature (39°C/102°F or above).

Aloe vera gel and lavender essential oil are two natural remedies for minor burns.

SUNSTROKE

A sunburned child may also develop heatstroke, with a raised temperature, headache, nausea, dizziness and general aches.

What to do. Cool your child down by sponging with tepid water. Give plenty of cool drinks to sip: water, diluted fruit juice or a rehydration drink (available from pharmacists). The homeopathic remedies Sol or Belladonna may be given.

When to seek help. Get immediate medical help if your child's temperature is very high (39°C/102°F).

FOREIGN OBJECTS IN THE EYE

Children can easily rub grit or other irritants into their eyes.

What to do. If you can see a piece of grit in your child's eye, get the child to put his or her head on one side with the affected side uppermost. Holding the eyelids open with your fingers, very slowly pour tepid water into the upper corner of the eye so that water covers the whole eye. If the grit doesn't move, try lifting it off with the corner of a damp handkerchief.

When to seek help. Seek immediate medical attention if something is stuck to the surface of the eye or embedded in it.

When your baby is sick

Babies can't tell you when they are sick, but as a parent you quickly become adept at reading the early signs. The first hint of illness is usually clinginess: your baby may want to be held all the time. This is a very natural response: the baby knows that something is wrong and wants you to take care of him or her. Babies are usually listless when they are ill: yours may be content to lie quietly in your arms and may be needing to sleep more than usual.

Other signs of illness include:

Looking unwell. A sick baby usually looks poorly, with a pathetic expression and dull eyes.

Reduced appetite. Sick babies tend to feed a lot less than normal: this won't harm your baby so long as he or she is taking enough fluid to prevent dehydration.

Irritability. Your baby may cry more than usual or in an unusual way. This can be a sign of pain.

Fever. Illness usually (but not always) goes hand-in-hand with a raised temperature, which causes babies to breathe more quickly than usual.

An unusual clinginess may be the first sign that your baby is ill. He or she instinctively knows that he needs to stay close to you.

WHEN TO SEEK HELP

It can be difficult to assess a baby's condition. Similar symptoms occur in serious and non-serious illnesses, and although symptoms are often more severe in a very sick baby, this is not always the case. It is best always to seek medical advice if you think your baby is ill, is refusing feeds or has unusual symptoms. Always see a doctor if a baby under three months has a fever.

Seek immediate medical help if your baby:

• has a seizure (fit)

• is limp and seems unaware of your presence

• is unusually drowsy and hard to wake up

• seems to be getting weaker or sicker by the hour

• is breathing very fast or noisily, or with difficulty, or if the skin between the ribs is sucked in as he or she breathes

• has a temperature over 39°C/102°F, especially if there is also a rash

• turns blue or becomes very pale, blotchy or ashen (if your baby is dark-skinned, check the palms)

• has a bulging or sunken fontanelle (the soft spot on the top of the head)

• has a purplish-red rash that doesn't disappear when you press a glass to it.

Rash. Skin rashes are a symptom of many illnesses and other conditions such as food sensitivity. Occasionally, they may have a serious cause, so it is essential to have an unexplained rash checked by a medical practitioner.

Diarrhoea and vomiting. Babies can be sick when they have an ear, chest or throat infection, and they may pass loose, smelly stools when they have a viral infection. Vomiting and diarrhoea occurring together usually indicate food poisoning or gastroenteritis.

TAKING YOUR BABY'S TEMPERATURE

A normal body temperature is 37°C/98.6°F, when taken by mouth. But it varies slightly depending on the time of day: a temperature taken in the morning will usually be slightly lower than one taken in the afternoon.

Poorly children need lots of fluids to prevent dehydration. A refreshing squeeze of lemon adds a little natural antiseptic to the drink.

A digital thermometer gives you an accurate reading of your child's temperature in an instant without your having to disturb him or her.

You can often tell that your child has a temperature simply by feeling the forehead. But it is best to get an accurate reading using a thermometer. Get a digital one that bleeps when an accurate reading has been taken: glass thermometers contain mercury, which is highly toxic if released into the atmosphere.

Under the arm. This is an easy way to take a baby's temperature. A normal temperature here is 36.4°C/97.4°F; anything over 37°C/98.6°F is a fever. Put your baby on your lap, place the thermometer under his or her arm and hold the arm against the baby's body to keep it in place.

Ear sensor. A digital ear thermometer takes a reading by measuring heat in the ear canal. It only takes a second and is not intrusive, but it is expensive.

Indicator strips. An indicator strip gives you the temperature of your baby's skin – not the body – so it is not an accurate measure.

CARING FOR A POORLY BABY
Sleep is a wonderful cure-all, and babies are naturally inclined to sleep more when poorly. But your baby

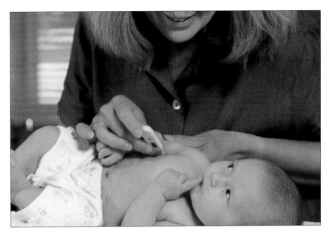

Using a digital thermometer under the arm is a safe and accurate method of reading your child's temperature.

probably won't want to be far from you. Be patient and keep the baby in your arms as much as possible: let the baby doze on you if that is what he or she needs. If your baby normally sleeps in a different room to you, then it is often a good idea to move the cot back in to your room so that you can monitor his or her condition more easily. Alternatively, sleep in the baby's room for a night or two.

Take steps to manage any fever and give frequent fluids to prevent dehydration: fever, diarrhoea, vomiting, coughing, crying or loss of appetite can all make your baby dehydrated. It's best to give fluids in small amounts to prevent your baby from vomiting it back up again. If you are breastfeeding, nurse often. Otherwise, give cooled, boiled water in addition to feeds (unless otherwise advised). If your baby is over six months, you can add a squeeze of lemon juice to the water – it has naturally antiseptic properties.

Don't feel that you have to keep your baby indoors: fresh air can be beneficial even if with a fever. Wrap the baby up well and go out for short periods.

Let a poorly child sleep as much as he or she needs: rest is one of the best natural medicines we have.

Common problems: colds, coughs and breathing disorders

Children get more coughs and colds than adults. Most children catch between six and eight colds a year until they build up immunity. And as the airways of a child are much smaller than those of adults, they are more vulnerable to infection.

COLDS

It is viruses that cause colds, so antibiotics do not help. A cold usually lasts a week or two, but can go on for longer in young children. Symptoms include a blocked-up or runny nose, sticky eyes, sore throat, a tickly cough (especially at night) and slight fever.

What to do. You can't hasten a cold's progress, but you can make your child more comfortable. Keep him or her warm, but open windows regularly to get fresh air circulating. Take your child out (well wrapped up) on short trips. Increase the humidity in the child's room to help with breathing: put a damp towel on the radiator, place a bowl of water near the radiator or other heat source or use a vaporizer.

Give lots of fluids. Children over a

For colds, give drinks of diluted blackcurrant, orange or lemon juice sweetened with a little honey.

year old can have hot honey and lemon, which is soothing for the throat and a good source of vitamin C. Weak elderflower tea acts as a decongestant. Dilute fruit juices can also be a good way of encouraging a child to drink. Unsweetened blackcurrant diluted with warm water is good if your child has a cold: it is packed with vitamin C.

- If your child is eating, cut out dairy products (which are mucus-forming) while symptoms remain, but give alternative sources of calcium such as tofu, ground nuts and seeds, and leafy green vegetables. Babies will still need their usual milk.
- Get older children to blow their nose regularly, to stop mucus dripping down the back of the throat.
- Consider giving a homeopathic remedy to soothe symptoms. The following are common cold remedies: Aconite, given in the first 24 hours; Allium cepa, when there is lots of watery discharge from the nose and eyes; Pulsatilla, when there is thick, greenish mucus

There are many homeopathic remedies for different types of cough and cold symptoms.

When to seek help. Seek medical advice if you spot other unusual signs, such as wheezing or earache, if the symptoms are very severe or if your child gets more poorly after a few days.

COUGHS

Coughing is how the body removes irritants or mucus from the breathing apparatus, so it is best to avoid over-the-counter medications that are designed to suppress this natural mechanism. If your child suddenly starts coughing violently, consider whether he or she may have inhaled a foreign object. Take steps to remove it from the airway (see first aid for choking).

What to do. If your child is coughing, the suggestions given for colds above are helpful, together with the following:

- Humidify all rooms by placing a bowl of water under the radiator or heat source.
- Avoid taking your child outdoors if the weather is cold and damp.
- For babies over three months, put a drop of essential oil of

Eucalyptus oil is a good natural decongestant, but you need only a drop on a tissue.

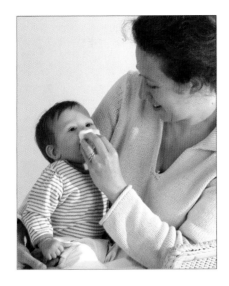

Use soft cotton wool (cotton balls) rather than tissues to wipe a child's nose to stop it getting sore.

eucalyptus smithi (not eucalyptus globulus, which is stronger) on a handkerchief and leave it in your child's room, out of reach.

- For children over one year, give diluted warm blackcurrant juice to soothe a sore throat, or thyme tea remedy (see box). If children are eating, include mild spices such as cinnamon or ginger in their food to help loosen mucus. Pineapple is also good because it contains bromeline, which is a natural anti-inflammatory.

- Consider giving one of the many homeopathic remedies used to relieve symptoms. A homeopath will help you pinpoint the right one for your child. Common remedies include: Aconite, for a dry cough that comes on at night; Bryonia, for a dry, painful cough (worse on inhalation) that follows a cold; Ipepac, for a cough that is accompanied by vomiting up phlegm; Phosphorus, for a dry, tickly cough that is worse at night; Pulsatilla, for a cough that produces yellow or green phlegm

When to seek help. Coughing can be a minor ailment or a symptom of some much more serious illnesses such as bronchiolitis and bronchitis. Always see a doctor if a cough occurs in a young baby, or if it is

severe, prolonged or accompanied by wheezing, noisy breathing or fast breathing.

CROUP

A barking cough and noisy breathing on inhalation are the key signs of croup, which is most common among children aged between six months and three years.

What to do. There are two ways to improve the breathing: take your child into a steamy room (run the hot shower and taps in the bathroom to create steam) or wrap the child up well and go outside into the cold air. Different approaches work for different children, so do which works best for your child.

THYME TEA REMEDY

This traditional remedy can help to ease a dry cough and loosen mucus. If possible, use New Zealand manuka honey, which has particular therapeutic properties.

Add a small handful of finely chopped thyme leaves to a cup of boiling water, steep until cool, then strain. Add honey to sweeten, then pour into a sterilized jar. Give 1 tsp three or four times a day. Keep in the refrigerator for up to 3 days.

For flu, try giving your child weak lime flower tea, which helps to treat fever and reduce nasal catarrh.

BRONCHIOLITIS

This viral infection is most common in babies under twelve months, and affects the smallest airways in the lungs (the bronchioles). It starts as a cold and fever and develops into coughing, fast breathing (more than 50 breaths a minute) and wheezing.

What to do. See your doctor quickly: sometimes hospital treatment is needed.

BRONCHITIS

This infection of the large airways (bronchi) is common in toddlers and children. The symptoms are similar to those of bronchiolitis. Deficiencies in vitamin C and zinc can be an underlying cause for recurrent lung problems such as bronchitis.

What to do. Medical advice should be sought. Giving a multivitamin multimineral supplement in addition may help.

FLU

The symptoms of flu include a high temperature, aches and pains, cold symptoms, vomiting and/or diarrhoea and general malaise.

What to do. See your doctor for a diagnosis. Lime flower and elderflower tea – or a combination of both – are good for flu. They should be drunk warm, well diluted.

Common problems: eczema, asthma and digestion

Asthma and eczema are now very common in young children. Both are the result of oversensitivity of the immune system, which cause it to react to substances that have no effect on other people. They often occur together, and affected children are also more likely to suffer from food allergies.

Nobody quite knows why asthma and eczema have become so prevalent, but it may be because improved living standards have reduced the amount of germs children come into contact with, with the result that their immune systems are less robust. The increase in pollution, outdoors and in, may also be a factor. Exclusive breastfeeding in the first months of life can reduce the likelihood of both asthma and eczema developing.

Babies have sensitive digestive systems that react quickly to get rid of unwanted substances: they are more prone to diarrhoea and vomiting than adults. These symptoms are the body's way of cleansing itself, so medications to stop them are generally unhelpful.

ECZEMA

There are different types of eczema: those that usually affect children are seborrhoeic eczema (cradle cap) and the itchy atopic eczema, which one child in five develops. Atopic eczema can affect any part of the body, but is most common on the face, armpits, elbows, hands and knees. During an acute attack, the skin reddens, becomes extremely itchy and can blister and weep. It may be thick, dry and flaky at other times.

What to do. See your doctor, as it's essential to manage your child's eczema to prevent infection. Eczema reduces the skin's ability to act as a barrier, and bacteria are more likely to stick to dry, flaky skin.

Avoid irritating the skin, choose clothing or bedding made from cotton, launder with non-biological washing powders, use half the amount you normally would, and use an extra rinse cycle on your washing machine. Don't use soap and bath products. Keep your child as cool as possible, as heat and sweating exacerbate eczema. Cut his or her fingernails short to help prevent scratching (put cotton mittens on babies and young children at night).

Keep your child's skin clean and moisturized. Give lukewarm (not hot) daily baths to remove dry skin scales and cleanse the skin. Use an emollient such as a handful of oatmeal tied in a muslin square (you can add a drop of lavender or chamomile essential oil). Different creams work for different children. Hemp seed oil cream is one good natural alternative to try, as is olive oil. Apply a thin layer and let it soak in rather than rubbing it in (which can increase itching).

Increase oils in your child's diet. Add a spoonful of hemp seed oil to your child's food each day and give

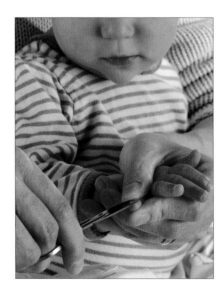

oily fish or a supplement. Give lots of water to keep your child well hydrated. Consider food sensitivity as an underlying factor, and see a qualified nutritional therapist to help you pinpoint any problem foods. Sugar can exacerbate eczema. A child-friendly probiotic will help to improve the balance of good bacteria in the gut, which can also be beneficial.

ASTHMA

Growing numbers of babies and children suffer from the attacks of breathlessness and wheezing that characterize asthma. Natural therapies can help to support conventional medical treatment.

What to do. Try to identify possible triggers for your child's asthma and take steps to avoid them. Your doctor can arrange tests to check for allergy to substances such as dust mites. Improve the air quality in your home and keep it free of dust (but vacuum when your child is out of the way). Choose a synthetic pillow and duvet with allergen-proof covers for your child's bed, and wash the bedding often in hot water. Limit toys in the cot to one or two, and wash them each week at 60°C/140°F or put in a plastic bag in the freezer overnight to kill dust mites.

Make sure that your child has a healthy diet including lots of fresh fruits and vegetables, and use organic produce wherever possible to reduce your child's exposure to pesticides. Do not put salt in your child's food, and avoid processed foods. Homeopathy may help. Arsenicum, Ipecac, Nat sulph and

Keep your child's fingernails short to stop him or her scratching areas of skin affected by eczema.

Olive oil mixed with chamomile and lavender essential oils may help with mild eczema symptoms.

Pulsatilla are all prescribed to relieve mild asthma attacks, but you should see a homeopath for a specific remedy for your baby. Herbal medicine has several remedies for asthma. A medical herbalist can advise you on the best herbs to use (alongside conventional treatment).

DIGESTIVE PROBLEMS

When a baby has diarrhoea, is sick or constipated, the best thing is to let it take its natural course. Your main aim should be to reduce discomfort and prevent dehydration.

Your child may get a short bout of diarrhoea (frequent, unpleasant-smelling, loose stools) after having a lot of fruit or fruit juice, after eating a food he or she is intolerant to, when teething or with a cold. A course of antibiotics can also sometimes be a trigger. Diarrhoea can be a sign of food poisoning or gastroenteritis, especially if accompanied by vomiting. In most cases, it lasts 24 hours or less and clears up by itself.
What to do. Give frequent drinks of water for sipping. Let a nursing baby

breastfeed on demand and give a bottle-fed baby extra drinks of cooled, boiled water. Antispasmodic herbal teas, such as chamomile or fennel, can ease tummy pains. Diluted unsweetened blackcurrant juice helps fight infection in the gut.

For a soothing tummy massage, add one drop chamomile essential oil to 15ml/1 tbsp olive or sunflower oil. Gently massage the tummy, with clockwise circular strokes.

Consider giving a suitable probiotic to help balance the bacteria in the gut. This can help reduce the duration of a bout of diarrhoea.
When to seek help. Contact a doctor if a baby has diarrhoea for more than a few hours. Seek medical help if the diarrhoea is severe, or there is blood in the stools, if your baby seems dehydrated or has persistent stomach ache or if he or she has taken something toxic.

Like diarrhoea, vomiting can have many causes. If your child is doing both, the most likely cause is gastroenteritis or food poisoning. Vomiting on its own can be the result of a baby having taken too much milk or can be part of a feverish illness. A baby with a cold may be sick, to expel phlegm from the body.
What to do. Treat as for diarrhoea (but avoid giving a tummy massage). Encourage your child to sip rather than to gulp liquid to help it stay down. Ginger is good for nausea: you can make a simple ginger tea by steeping a block of peeled, bruised ginger in a cup of hot water.
When to seek help. Contact your doctor if a baby vomits repeatedly or violently, or if vomiting and diarrhoea occur together.

If your child suddenly goes for longer than normal between bowel movements, and then produces hard, dry, pebble-like stools, he or she is constipated.
What to do. Increase the vegetables and fruits in your child's diet (but cut out bananas): broccoli, leafy green

vegetables and dried apricots are particularly helpful. Most important of all, make sure your baby is well hydrated: give extra water.

Flaxseeds are rich in fibre and are a natural lubricant. Consider putting 5ml/1 tsp flaxseed oil into a fruit smoothie. Give live yoghurt if the balance of the intestinal flora has been upset by a bout of gastroenteritis or a course of antibiotics. Or consider giving a child-friendly probiotic supplement.

Massage can soothe cramping and encourage the bowels to move: stroke your hand over the abdomen, making an arch shape in a clockwise direction so that you are following the line of the intestines. If constipation is a recurring problem, consider whether food sensitivity could be a root cause. An Italian study found that sensitivity to cow's milk caused chronic constipation in some children.
When to seek help. Seek medical advice if your child does not have a bowel movement for several days, or if the problem is recurrent.

A probiotic drink for children may help with digestive problems.

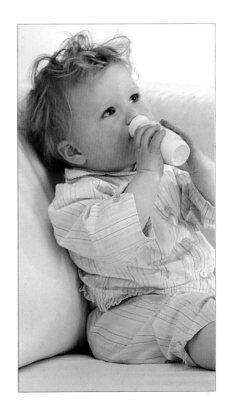

Common problems: skin rashes and ear infections

Rashes are a feature of many childhood infections, both non-serious and serious. It's quite hard to distinguish between different rashes, so it is best to check them out with your doctor.

CHICKENPOX

The first symptoms of chickenpox are usually tiredness, fever and loss of appetite. Within a day or two, small, flat red spots appear, usually on the back, stomach and chest. They can spread to the face and head in a day or two. The red spots join up and blister, becoming intensely itchy. They scab over within 24 hours, as more spots appear.

Chickenpox is infectious from two days before the spots appear until scabs have formed on all the spots. It takes 10–21 days for the symptoms to appear after infection. One attack usually confers lifelong immunity. Chickenpox can be very dangerous for unborn children if the mother is not immune, so if your child has been in contact with a pregnant woman, let her know, so that she can contact her doctor.

Chickenpox spots blister and then scab. They are itchy, but discourage your child from scratching in case of infection and scarring.

Make an elderflower infusion, dip cotton wool in the bowl and dab on the spots for relief from itching.

What to do. Encourage your child to rest as much as possible and take steps to manage any fever. Use calendula cream or calomine lotion on the spots to relieve itching, or dab them with elderflower tea or a solution of 5ml/1 tsp distilled witch hazel in a cup of warm water. Give lots of fruits and vegetables to boost your child's immune system, and add raw garlic to food if your child will eat it. Consider giving the following homeopathic remedies:

- Aconite, for the initial symptoms of tiredness and fever
- Belladonna, for the early stages if temperature is high and the child is flushed and very thirsty
- Rhus tox, for itching and any restlessness

Encourage your child to eat lots of healthy fruits and vegetables to promote healing.

Protect your child's skin from direct sunlight for a couple of weeks after the scabs fall off, to avoid any danger of scarring.

When to seek help. See your doctor if a baby is affected, if the attack is severe, if the spots become inflamed or if you are pregnant and are not sure that you are immune.

HEAT RASH

Young children have immature sweat glands, which are easily blocked. Heat rash usually appears as small red bumps, sometimes with a blister in the centre, that appear on areas exposed to sunlight or areas that sweat a lot.

What to do. Cool your child down: remove clothing, sponge down or give the child a tepid bath. Good topical treatments include aloe vera gel, distilled witch hazel, Calendula cream or a lavender or chamomile compress. The homeopathic remedy Sol can also be helpful.

IMPETIGO

This infectious skin condition usually starts off around the mouth or nose. It takes the form of red blisters, which soon burst and form a golden crust on reddened, weeping skin.

RELIEVING ITCHING CHICKENPOX SPOTS
A lukewarm oatmeal bath can be soothing. Place a handful of oatmeal in a muslin square or the foot of a nylon stocking, add 2 drops each of chamomile and lavender essential oils, tie up and place in the water. Give several baths a day.

GLUE EAR

This is a condition in which thick, sticky fluid accumulates in the middle ear, leading to hearing problems. It can be linked to repeated ear or throat infections, which block the Eustachian tube. If it is persistent, the conventional treatment is the insertion of a plastic grommet to allow fluid to drain. But the procedure involves a general anaesthetic and has itself been linked to hearing problems. Repeated ear infections are often a cause, so take steps to avoid them (see above). Many complementary health practitioners believe that glue ear is linked to food sensitivity, particularly an intolerance of dairy foods, or to passive smoking.

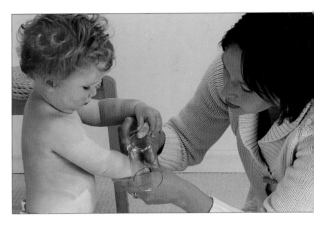

What to do. Bathing the skin with warm salt water can help to reduce itching; tea tree oil added neat to water can also help with itching and can limit the infection. Give garlic perles every two hours for a day or two, then reduce to three times a day, to help resolve the infection. The homeopathic remedies Ant crud or Arsenicum can be useful.

Be scrupulous about hygiene: do not share face towels or pillows and keep your child away from other children while infectious.

EAR INFECTIONS

Children are prone to ear infections, particularly after a cold or throat infection. The Eustachian tube, the drainage canal that links the nose, ear and throat, is very narrow. If it becomes blocked, fluid accumulates and viruses and bacteria multiply. The main symptoms are pain, hearing loss and fever. A small child

Warmth can soothe the pain of an earache; use a covered hot water bottle or a lavender compress.

may tug on the ear, but most simply cry and seem unwell.

Seek medical advice straight away if you suspect your child has an ear infection. It needs prompt treatment – usually antibiotics – to prevent the infection spreading. Take steps to prevent recurrence, so your child does not have to take repeated courses of antibiotics.

What you can do. Warm the affected ear by holding a warm lavender compress or a covered hot-water bottle against it. Dilute lavender essential oil in olive or sunflower oil and smooth into the skin around the ear and neck.

For children over one year, give plenty of warm drinks such as honey and lemon and fresh blackcurrant juice; you can give a herbal tea combining chamomile (antiseptic and relaxing), elderflower or lemon balm (to reduce mucus) and lime flowers (to bring down fever) three times a day. Garlic can help relieve infection: add fresh garlic to your child's food if possible, or give garlic perles. If your child has taken antibiotics, give live yoghurt every day for a month to help rebalance the bacteria in the gut.

Raise the head of the cot or bed to help fluid drain from the Eustachian tube. Avoid washing your child's hair or going swimming while symptoms persist. Consider giving a homeopathic remedy, such as:

- Aconite, at the onset of symptoms, especially if the child has a blocked nose, fever and is thirsty
- Belladonna, for earache that is

To test for a meningitis rash, press a clear glass against it, if the spots do not disappear seek immediate medical aid.

worse at night and better when the child sits upright
- Chamomilia, for earache that accompanies teething, is causing extreme pain and irritability
- Pulsatilla, for earache with a cold that is worse at night.

If your child gets repeated ear infections, keep his or her ears, throat and neck warm at all times: wrap the child up well in cold weather. Give the remedies mentioned above at the first signs of a cold, to try to head off infections, but seek advice from a homeopath for a remedy specifically tailored to your child. Consider food sensitivity as a possible cause. Dairy products are the most common culprits, but wheat, eggs and chocolate could also be triggers in some children.

Make sure your child is eating a healthy, balanced diet, with plenty of fresh fruits and vegetables, zinc-rich foods such as meat and poultry, and lots of garlic. Do not give sugar, which depresses the immune system. Warm drinks of honey and lemon or diluted fresh blackcurrant juice support the immune system and encourage mucus to clear. Consider giving a multivitamin, multimineral supplement.

When to seek help. See a doctor if you suspect an ear infection, or if blood or clear liquid is discharged from the ear.

A healthy home

We are all exposed to toxic chemicals every day: they are in the air we breathe, our food and drink and the toiletries and household products we use. Because our homes are enclosed spaces, toxin levels can build up and the air can actually be more polluted than it is outdoors. Ordinary household dust can contain a mixture of solvents, hormone-disrupting chemicals, heavy metals, solvents, pesticides and flame retardants. Babies spend a lot of their time indoors and they are more likely to be affected by pollution than adults. So it is important to ensure that your home is a healthy environment for your child to grow up in.

Here are some basic steps for a healthy home.
- Ban smoking at home.
- Open your windows regularly.
- Keep pets out of sleeping areas. If your child is allergic to your pet, you may have to keep it out of all living areas or find it a new home.
- Wipe your feet when you come in, and leave your shoes by the door to avoid bringing dirt, heavy metals and toxic chemicals indoors.
- Choose furniture made from untreated natural materials.
- Wash curtains, other soft furnishings and bedclothes regularly.

Keeping your home dust-free will help to protect your baby from inhaling pollutants. But use natural products rather than spray polishes and carpet cleaners.

NATURAL CLEANING PRODUCTS

You can use ordinary ingredients to tackle many cleaning jobs around the home.

Bicarbonate of soda (baking soda). Sprinkle this on a damp sponge and use to clean surfaces. For stubborn stains, mix it with a little water and leave for 20 minutes before wiping off. Add 30ml/2 tbsp bicarbonate of soda to a cup of vinegar and add to the toilet bowl. Leave for at least 15 minutes, then clean with a brush. To clean a drain, add half a cup of bicarbonate then half a cup of vinegar. Leave for 15 minutes, then pour down a kettle of boiling water.

White vinegar. This is great for cleaning windows. Add half a cup of vinegar to 1 litre/2 pints warm water and apply with a soft cloth, then buff with crumpled newspaper. Vinegar can also be used for descaling appliances: add equal parts of vinegar and water to a kettle and leave overnight. Throw out the vinegar, boil the kettle and discard the water before using again.

Lemon juice. Lemon is an excellent natural brightening agent and cleanser. Add half a cup of lemon juice to a bucket of water and soak white or coloured clothes overnight before washing as usual.

- Keep your home as dust-free as possible. Consider buying a vacuum cleaner with a high-efficiency particulate air (HEPA) filter. Keep children out of the way while you dust and vacuum.
- Dry clothes outside or in a properly ventilated space. Avoid putting them around the house (on radiators and so on); the moisture will be released into the air and may cause the growth of mould spores in your walls.

DECORATING

If you are planning a nursery for your baby or revamping a child's bedroom, seek out non-toxic decorating products and furnishings. Babies and children spend a lot of time on or near the floor, so choose a natural covering such as wood or cork rather than laminate or vinyl, which may contain harmful chemicals. Hard flooring is the best option because carpet traps dust, which can lead to a build-up of airborne toxins and dust mites. But if you want to use carpet for warmth, choose wool, sisal or coir with a natural backing, and vacuum regularly.

Regular paints contain volatile organic compounds (VOCs), which give off noxious vapours after being applied. Choose water-based low-VOC paints, keep the room well ventilated during and after decorating and don't let your baby sleep in the room for a few days after painting it. Better still, use organic paints made from natural materials such as linseed, casein and mineral pigments. These take longer to dry and can be harder to use, but they are safe for allergy- and asthma-sufferers.

If you are picking furniture for a baby's room, avoid items made from MDF, laminated wood or chipboard, which contain formaldehyde. Choose furniture made from untreated hardwood from sustainable sources instead. Use natural materials for your baby's bedding. For example, get a mattress made from organic latex, wool and cotton, and sheets of unbleached organic cotton.

CUT THE CHEMICALS

Reducing the amount of chemicals you use in the home will lower the risk of your baby coming into contact with something harmful.

- If your kitchen cupboard is a jumble of different products, go through it and get rid of any products you don't use. General cleaners may leave a residue on your surfaces, which your baby may then touch: so avoid those labelled 'irritant' and choose gentle eco-friendly products or natural cleaning alternatives instead.

Young children inevitably spend a lot of time on the floor, so it is worth investing in natural coverings that are free from unnecessary chemicals.

- In the same way, go through your bathroom cupboards and throw out any products that you do not need. Avoid wearing perfume, hairspray and a plethora of other products to reduce the amount of chemicals your baby breathes in. He or she will prefer your natural smell in any case. Put only natural substances on your baby or toddler – he or she can do without bubble baths, wipes, talc and harsh soaps.

- Get rid of garden pesticides, weed killers and so on. Many common garden products – including creosote – have now been banned, so it is best to dispose of any products you have had for several years. Consider gardening organically to help protect your child from hazardous chemicals. For example, use saucers of beer sunk into the soil to trap slugs rather than poisonous pellets (which a young child could eat).

Left: Avoid using unnecessary toiletries. Many bubble baths contain detergent, which irritates the skin, while the ingredients for baby wipes may include propylene glycol – a chemical that is also present in anti-freeze.

Right: Make sure your child spends some time outside every day, whatever the weather.

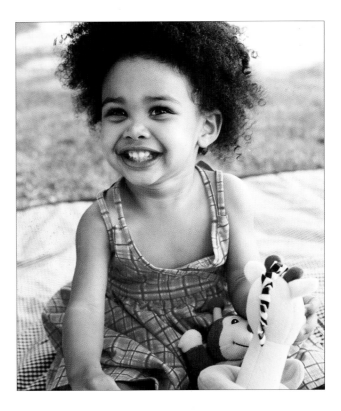

Safety when you are out

However safe you make your own home, you are bound to take your children to other people's homes that are less child-friendly. Get in the habit of scanning any room your child enters for possible hazards. Most people won't mind if you ask them to move something breakable from your child's reach or to move their coffee cup from the corner of a table. Be careful around animals that are unused to children: err on the side of caution and keep your child well away. If you plan to leave your child in another person's care, make sure that you are happy the environment is safe enough – don't leave your child if you are worried.

Be extra vigilant if there is a pond: about 80 per cent of drownings in garden ponds happen when children are visiting friends or relatives. If you go to a park where there is a pond or lake, keep very close to your child.

CAR JOURNEYS

All children should be fastened into properly fitted car seats for car journeys, however short. Never be tempted to take a trip holding your child in your lap; you will not be able to hold on to the child if your car is hit, and you could injure him or her with your body on impact.

Choose a car seat that meets recognized safety standards, and check with the manufacturer that it is suitable for your particular car. Don't buy a second-hand car seat: you won't know if it has been weakened in a previous accident, and it may have been made to less rigorous safety standards than a new seat.

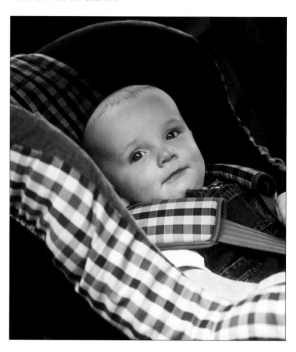

WHICH CAR SEAT?

Babies (Group 0): Rear-facing seats are needed for babies from birth to 10–13kg/22–29lb. But it is best to avoid taking a very young baby on a long car journey if you can. Keep your baby in this first car seat until he or she outgrows it.

Older babies and toddlers (Group 1): Forward-facing seats are suitable for children from about nine months (so long as they can sit up well unsupported and weigh at least 9kg/20lb). They last until the child is about four and weighs 18kg/40lb.

Young children (Group 2): Booster seats are suitable for children weighing 15–25kg/33–55lb, usually between the ages of four and six. Like car seats for younger children, they are best fitted in the back of the car rather than the front, and this is essential if there is an airbag in the front of the car. They don't have a separate harness as car seats do; instead the seatbelt goes around both the seat and the child.

Older children (Group 3): Children should use some sort of booster seat until they reach the age of 11. Booster cushions are used for children weighing 22–36kg/48–79lb.

Children are instinctively drawn by water. Never leave your child unattended in a garden with a pond; keep him or her in sight at all times.

Around 10 minutes of sun early or late in the day helps your child to make essential vitamin D. But he or she needs a high-factor suncream at other times.

Many car seats are fitted incorrectly, so go to a specialist if you need help. If your car is new, go for an ISOFIX car seat, which is much easier to fit.

- Never fit a car seat in the front seat of a car if there is an airbag in front of it – the airbag could seriously harm (and possibly kill) your child if it inflates. It is safer to fit the seat in the back even if there is no airbag.
- Make sure that the seat belt goes through all guides on the seat.
- Check the seat belt is pulled tight before every journey: the seat shouldn't rock sideways or forwards when you try to move it.
- Don't have the buckle of the seatbelt resting on the frame of the car seat; it could snap open in an accident.
- Adjust the harness so it fits snugly. Check it at the start of every journey, as the fit will depend on what your child is wearing. Don't have the buckle resting on your child's tummy.
- If you are using a booster seat, make sure the seatbelt rests against your child's shoulder, not his neck, and from hip bone to hip bone.

OUT IN THE SUN

Children's skin is thinner than adults', so you need to be vigilant about protecting it from sunburn: damage to the skin now could have long-term effects. Babies under six months should be kept out of direct sunlight entirely. If your baby is in a buggy or pram, use a UV sunshade. If you are carrying a baby in a sling, cover his or her arms and legs with a light but closely woven fabric such as cotton and get a wide-brimmed hat.

SUN FOODS
Foods containing the antioxidant beta-carotene may help protect the skin from the harmful effects of the sun. Carrots, melons, mango, apricots and spinach are all good sources that are worth including in your child's summer diet.

Put sunscreen on the baby's hands and feet if they are exposed. Older babies and young children should be kept out of direct sunlight as much as possible during the hottest part of the day (10am–4pm on very hot days). Apply a high-factor sunscreen at least half an hour before you go outside. Use a sunscreen made from natural ingredients with an SPF of at least 20. This will be gentler on your child's skin than very high factor sunscreens that last three or four hours (but which may get rubbed off beforehand in any case). Apply a thick layer and let it sink into the skin rather than rubbing in. Reapply frequently. However, if you know that your child is going to be out in the sun for some time, especially in someone else's care, use a higher factor to be on the safe side. Remember that skin can still burn on warm cloudy days, or in the shade next to water or sand, which reflects sunlight.

Your child will need more fluids when it is hot. If you are breastfeeding, nurse frequently: your milk has a higher water content on hot days so your baby shouldn't need extra drinks.

Some children refuse to hold hands when they are out and about – in which case you will need reins or a wrist strap to keep them safe.

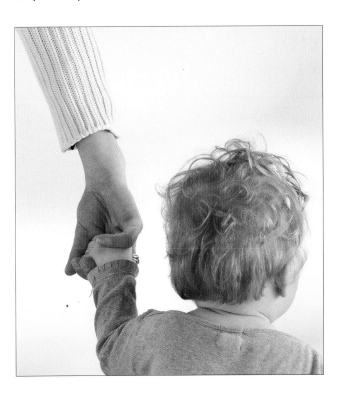

Meal planning for babies

First foods should be easy for babies to eat and digest, so baby rice, puréed root vegetables and pears and apples are ideal, but there is no strict rule about exactly which foods to give first, so it is fine if you want to chop and change. However, do make sure you don't introduce any foods that may cause an allergic reaction until the ages recommended in Chapter 5. The menu planner on the opposite page starts at six months: if you are starting solids earlier, you will have to adapt it slightly so that you don't introduce foods such as chicken, fish or wheat too early.

INTRODUCING SOLIDS

It helps your baby to adjust to new flavours if you mix each food with his or her usual milk or with milky baby rice for the first few times you give it.

FOOD PLANNER
This planner will help you when introducing your baby to solid food. It suggests which foods to introduce when, but remember that each week you will be adding a different food, not feeding your baby only that one, so by week 4, for example, you will be trying baby rice, carrot, squash and pear.

Week	Introduce
1	baby rice
2	carrot
3	squash or swede (rutabaga)
4	pear
5	parsnip, apple
6	banana, potato, rice cakes
7	courgette (zucchini), mango, melon
8	green beans, nectarine/peach
9	natural yoghurt, red lentils
10	leeks, chicken, cauliflower
11	oats, cheese
12	white fish, grain such as quinoa, polenta or millet
13	pasta, onions, grapes
14	bread, lamb
15	beans, spinach
16	apricots, celery, sweet (bell) peppers
17	tomatoes, salmon
18	aubergine (eggplant), mushrooms
19	peas, egg yolk
20	tofu or beef, citrus fruit (such as mandarins)

Giving fruits and vegetables of different colours will help your child to get a good range of vitamins.

Meat, eggs, tomatoes and citrus fruits can be introduced once the baby is well established on solids.

You can gradually introduce a wider variety of fruits and vegetables to your child.

Babies like sweet tastes, so root vegetables, pears and apples mixed with baby rice are good first foods.

Alternate the new food with foods you have already introduced, so that your baby gets used to having different tastes at every meal. You can combine purées, too, mixing squash and carrot, carrot and parsnip, parsnip and apple and so on. Be sure to leave three days before introducing each new food, to allow time for any reaction to show itself. However, once your baby is eating lots of different foods, you can introduce a flavouring such as garlic at the same time as, say, lentils. Remember that you shouldn't cut down on milk feeds until the end of the first year.

PLANNING YOUR MENUS
Once you have a few meals prepared and stored in the freezer, it's easy to give your baby a good and varied diet. Pasta or rice with butter, cheese and a few chopped

Grains are an important source of energy, while chicken, pulses and dairy foods are good protein foods.

vegetables mixed in, or mashed avocado, make a good quick meal if you run out. Your baby may need a few snacks as well as the usual milk in between meals. Use the menu planner as a guide, and remember that so long as you vary foods throughout a week, your baby will be getting a good mix of nutrients, even if on one day they refuse to eat anything other than grapes.

Breastfed babies will usually have more milk feeds, but a routine might look like this:

A good quick meal is rice with a spoonful of cooked vegetables and some grated cheese.

On waking Milk, then breakfast
11.30 am Lunch with water
2.30 pm Milk and afternoon snack
5.00 pm Supper with water
7.00 pm Milk

MENU PLANNER FOR A BABY FROM NINE TO TWELVE MONTHS

Adapt this to your needs and routine and vary it if you need to.

Day 1
Breakfast Oat porridge with banana
Lunch Tarragon chicken with potatoes
   Plain yoghurt
Snack Pear slices and toast fingers
Supper Vegetable soup with rice

Day 2
Breakfast Oat/millet porridge with pear purée
   Toast fingers
Lunch Lentil dhal with rice or quinoa and spinach
Snack Rice cakes and apple slices
Supper Pasta with peas, olive oil and cheese
   Mango purée

Day 3
Breakfast Wheat biscuit cereal with banana
Lunch Cauliflower and broccoli cheese
   Raspberry and apple purée
Snack Polenta fingers and pear slices
Supper Fish pilau

Day 4
Breakfast Oat porridge with mango and cinnamon
   Toast fingers
Lunch Beany bake
Snack Rice cakes, grapes
Supper Buttery rice with swede (rutabaga) purée and broccoli
   Natural yoghurt with fruit purée

Day 5
Breakfast Millet porridge with pear and banana
Lunch Ratatouille with pitta fingers
   Strawberries or raspberries with

Greek yoghurt
Snack Oatcakes and melon chunks
Supper Lamb casserole with rice

Day 6
Breakfast Wheat biscuit cereal with pear
Lunch Poached salmon with rice, sugar snap peas and cooked tomato
Snack Banana
Supper Vegetable soup and mini cream cheese sandwiches (add pineapple to the cheese and blend to a purée)

Day 7
Breakfast Oat porridge with banana
Lunch Couscous salad
   Apricot compote
Snack Polenta fingers and grapes
Supper Lightly fried chicken fillet, rice and steamed carrot sticks

Recipes for babies: six to nine months

Once your baby is eating a range of foods, you can start combining ingredients to make more interesting meals. Here are some suggestions for easy-to-cook, baby-friendly dishes.

BABY RICE

It's worth making your own baby rice once your baby is eating more than a couple of teaspoonfuls at a time. You won't get it as smooth as the commercial variety, but this is a good way to start introducing texture. Use white rice not brown.

50g/2oz white rice
Breast or formula milk

Bring a small saucepan of water to the boil, add the rice and stir once. Leave to simmer for about 10 minutes, until the rice grains are tender. Drain the rice, then purée with your baby's usual milk.

COURGETTE PURÉE

Steamed courgettes (zucchini) go well with sweet carrots. Leave the skin on the carrot if it is organic.

1 courgette
1 carrot

Chop the courgette and peel and chop the carrot. Put the carrot in a steamer and cook for 5 minutes. Add the courgette and steam for another 10 minutes, until both vegetables are very soft. Purée with your baby's usual milk or use a little of the water used to steam the vegetables.

POTATO, SWEDE AND SWEET POTATO MASH

Root vegetables purée well and have a nice sweet taste. You can add a pinch of garam masala to the combination to liven it up once your baby is well established on solid foods and ready for new tastes.

2 large potatoes
Quarter of a small swede (rutabaga)
1 small sweet potato

Peel and dice all the vegetables and steam them for 15–20 minutes, until soft. Blend or mash with your baby's usual milk until smooth.

CHICKEN, PARSNIP AND GREEN BEAN PURÉE

Any vegetable purée goes well with chicken, but parsnip has a wonderfully sweet taste that babies love. Use broccoli or leeks in place of the beans if you like.

1 parsnip
50g/2oz fine green beans
1 small chicken breast
A little olive oil, for frying

Cut the parsnip into quarters lengthways. Cut out the woody core from each piece then chop into small chunks. Top and tail the beans. Steam the parsnip for 5 minutes then add the green beans to the steamer and continue cooking for another 10 minutes, until are soft.

Meanwhile, cut the chicken breast into small pieces. Heat a little olive oil in a frying pan, and fry the chicken for 6–7 minutes until cooked through. Combine the cooked chicken with the vegetables and blend or mash until smooth.

VEGETABLE SOUP

Soup slips down easily, so it is great for times when your baby is tired and doesn't want to eat much. This is a simple recipe that you can also use as a pasta sauce. Substitute celery for the leeks if you like, but in this case add half a chopped onion to the pan and fry for 2–3 minutes before adding the other vegetables.

STOCK

Most commercial stocks are too salty for babies. Good supermarkets and health food stores stock low-salt, good-quality bouillon, but, better still, make your own – it's pretty easy and once you get into the habit of doing it you won't want to go back to cubes. Store stock in the refrigerator for up to 4 days or freeze for up to 3 months.

For vegetable stock

Chop 1 celery stick, 1 large carrot, 1 large leek, 1 onion and 1 garlic clove. Put in a pan with 5 peppercorns, 2 sprigs of parsley (or parsley stalks), 2 sprigs of thyme and a bay leaf. Cover with 1.2 litres/2 pints/5 cups water, and bring to the boil. Skim off any froth, cover the pan, reduce the heat and simmer for 45 minutes. Leave to cool. Pour through a sieve lined with muslin (a baby muslin is ideal).

For chicken stock

Break up the carcass of a cooked chicken. Chop 1 onion, 1 carrot and 1 celery stick and place in a pan with the chicken bones, 5 peppercorns, 2 cloves, a small handful of parsley (or parsley stalks) and a bay leaf. Cover with 1.2 litres/2 pints/5 cups water, and bring to the boil. Skim off any froth, cover the pan, reduce the heat and simmer for 1 hour. Fish out the big bones, then strain through a muslin-lined sieve.

2 medium leeks, cleaned
4 large potatoes
2 carrots
A little olive oil, for frying
1.2 litres/2 pints/5 cups vegetable stock
Handful of parsley, finely chopped

Slice the leeks. Cut the potatoes into large chunks, and peel (unless organic) and slice the carrots.

Put a little olive oil in a pan over a low heat and add the vegetables. Cook for 5 minutes, stirring all the time. Add the stock, bring to a simmer, cover and cook for 25 minutes. Add the parsley and cook for 5 minutes, then blend.

LENTIL DHAL

Babies love dhal. You can purée this one with a serving of baby rice and some sliced cooked spinach to make a balanced meal in one – it's good with a spoonful of bio-active yoghurt. You can also add a spoonful of dhal to vegetable soup to make it a more substantial meal.

50g/2oz red lentils, washed
Small slice of ginger
Half a clove of garlic (sliced lengthways)
1 bay leaf
1 tomato (optional)

Place the lentils in a small pan. Pour in water up to a level about one and a half times the depth of the lentils. Add the ginger, garlic and bay leaf.

Bring to the boil, skim off any froth, reduce the heat, cover the pan and simmer for about 25 minutes or until the lentils are very tender.

Meanwhile, pour boiling water over the tomato, if using. Leave for a minute or two, remove the skin, cut in half, deseed and chop finely.

When the lentils are soft, discard the ginger and bay leaf, but mash the garlic into the dhal. Add the chopped tomato, if using, and cook for another 5 minutes. Blend if your baby is still eating smooth purées.

Variation: For a spicier dhal, fry half an onion in vegetable oil. Add 1.5ml/ $1/_4$ tsp each of ground coriander and ground cumin and fry for a further minute or two. Add this to the dhal.

RASPBERRY AND APPLE PURÉE

Simple fruit purées are a great way of getting vitamins into your baby.

1 eating apple, peeled and diced
115g/4oz raspberries

Place the fruit in a small pan with a tablespoon of water. Cook over a low heat for 5 minutes, or until soft. Purée the fruit, then pass through a sieve to remove the seeds.

APRICOT COMPOTE

3 ready-to-eat dried apricots
1 eating apple, peeled and diced
1 large nectarine, stoned

Chop the apricots and nectarine. Place all the fruits in a small pan with a little water. Simmer for about 10 minutes, until very soft, then purée.

Recipes for babies: nine to twelve months

Once you have introduced a reasonable number of different foods, cooking for your baby becomes a lot more fun. Here are some baby-friendly meals that older children (and adults) will love too.

CAULIFLOWER AND BROCCOLI CHEESE

You can add this cheese sauce to any cooked vegetables, or pasta. Use formula or full-fat cow's milk, and choose a cheese with a good flavour – babies like stronger tastes than you might think.

1 small cauliflower, in florets
1 head of broccoli, in florets

For the cheese sauce:
50g/2oz butter
20ml/1 rounded tbsp flour
300ml/½ pint/1¼ cups full-fat milk
115g/4oz Cheddar cheese,
  grated
Dab of English mustard (enough
  to cover the tip of a teaspoon)
Pinch of cayenne pepper

Steam the vegetables for about 10–12 minutes until soft.

Meanwhile, to make the sauce, melt the butter in a small pan. Stir in the flour for 1 minute, until the flour is completely cooked. Very slowly pour in the milk, stirring all the time. It will go into a lump at first, but keep stirring and adding the milk slowly. Bring the mixture slowly to the boil, then take the pan off the heat. Add the cheese, mustard and cayenne pepper. Keep stirring.

Add the sauce to the vegetables. Purée in a blender or mash well with a fork, depending on the age of your baby. If you are cooking for an older child, leave the florets whole.

TARRAGON CHICKEN

If you are bringing your child up to eat meat, chicken is likely to figure often on the menu. This easy stew contains leeks and mushrooms, but you can add other vegetables as well. Choose organic chicken.

2 large chicken breast fillets
2 medium leeks, washed
A little vegetable oil, for frying
Knob of butter
450ml/¾ pint/2 cups stock, or
  to cover
Handful of parsley, chopped
1 sprig fresh tarragon (or a large
  pinch of dried tarragon)
450g/1lb large flat mushrooms
5ml/1 tsp cornflour
Freshly ground black pepper

Cut the chicken into small chunks. Finely chop the leeks.

Heat the vegetable oil in a flameproof casserole or a deep heavy-bottomed frying pan. Fry the chicken in two or three batches over a medium heat for 6–7 minutes, until cooked through. Set aside.

Add the butter to the same pan and cook the leeks for 6–7 minutes until softened but not browned. Return the chicken to the pan. Add the stock and season with a couple of twists of black pepper. Add the herbs and leave to simmer for 10 minutes, uncovered, stirring from time to time, until slightly reduced. Chop the mushrooms very small and add to the pan. Cook for a further 6–7 minutes until cooked down.

When the stew is cooked, put about 50ml/2 fl oz/¼ cup water in a cup. Sprinkle in the cornflour and stir until dissolved. Add the mixture to the stew and cook for a further 2–3 minutes to thicken the sauce.

Variation: You can add 450g/1lb new potatoes, chopped into small dice, to the stew to make a complete meal. If you want to add more vegetables, try half a green (bell) pepper or a large carrot, diced. Cook the potatoes and the extra vegetables with the leeks.

LAMB CASSEROLE

Red meat is the best source of iron, so it is good to include it in your child's diet. Lamb is the first red meat to introduce to your baby: it is very easy to digest and most babies love it. Make sure you choose lean minced (ground) lamb, or trim the meat and mince it yourself, as lamb can be fatty. Choose organic meat if you can.

A little vegetable oil, for frying
450g/1lb minced (ground) lamb
1 large onion, finely chopped
2 large carrots, diced
2 courgettes (zucchini), diced
225g/½lb mushrooms, diced
300ml/½ pints/1¼ cups vegetable stock
400g/14oz can chopped tomatoes
5ml/1 tsp tomato purée
Pinch of mixed herbs
5ml/1 tsp cornflour

Heat a little vegetable oil in a flameproof casserole or a deep, heavy-bottomed frying pan. Brown the meat in two or three batches for about 5 minutes over a high heat. Set aside.

Lower the heat under the pan and add the chopped onion and carrot. Cook for 5–6 minutes, until softened. Add the courgettes and mushrooms and cook until soft.

Return the meat to the pan, then pour over the stock. Stir in the canned tomatoes, the tomato purée and the herbs. Cover and simmer for 40 minutes. Stir from time to time.

Put about 50ml/2 fl oz/¼ cup water in a cup. Sprinkle in the cornflour and stir until dissolved.

Add the mixture to the stew and cook for a further 2–3 minutes to thicken the sauce.

SIMPLE FISH PILAU

This is a simple fish dish that you can make just as easily with salmon.

200g/7oz cod or haddock fillet
Milk to cover
1 onion, finely chopped
2 garlic cloves, crushed
A little olive oil, for frying
Knob of butter
200g/7oz basmati rice
600ml/1 pint/2½ cups vegetable or fish stock
225g/8oz tomatoes
50g/2oz frozen peas
Small handful of parsley, chopped
Freshly ground black pepper

Place the fish in a small pan and cover with milk. Cook on a low heat until the fish is just opaque – about 5–7 minutes.

Heat a little olive oil in a frying pan. Add the onion and garlic and sweat for 6–7 minutes, until softened but not browned. Add the butter to the pan and let it melt, then add the rice, and stir until coated. Pour in half the stock and stir until it is absorbed into the rice, then add the rest a little at a time until the rice is cooked (about 25 minutes). Skin and deseed the tomatoes and chop, add with the peas to the rice mixture, and cook for a further 5 minutes.

Flake the cooked fish, removing any bones, and add to the rice with the herbs. Season with a twist of black pepper, and cook the pilau for a further 2–3 minutes, stirring.

RATATOUILLE

This is great with mashed potato, rice or buttery pasta.

Half a small onion, chopped
A little olive oil, for frying
1 clove garlic, chopped
1 red (bell) pepper, diced
2 courgettes (zucchini), diced
1 aubergine (eggplant), diced
2 large mushrooms, diced
4 tomatoes, peeled and chopped
5ml/1 tsp sun-dried tomato paste
Small handful of basil, chopped

Pour a little olive oil into a frying pan over a low heat and fry the onion for 6–7 minutes, until softened. Add the garlic, pepper, courgette, aubergine and mushrooms and cook for 7–8 minutes. Add the tomatoes, tomato paste and herbs. Cook for a further 15 minutes, uncovered, stirring gently from time to time.

FOOD ON THE GO

Sticks of cheese, mini sandwiches, easy-to-eat fruit or small pots of natural yoghurt are all ideal foods to take out with you. For a more substantial lunch, you could make an easy couscous or pasta salad.

Couscous salad

Pour a serving of couscous into a teacup and cover with boiling water. Add 5ml/1 tsp olive oil, cover and leave for 3–4 minutes for the grains to swell. Cook a few peas, and a chopped tomato in a pan with a tiny amount of water. Add to the couscous with some Cheddar cheese cut into tiny dice.

Pasta salad

Combine some cooked pasta shapes with some finely diced, cooked carrots and peas, flaked canned tuna, chopped parsley and a little olive oil.

Useful contacts

UK
Association of Breastfeeding Mothers
PO Box 207, Bridgewater
TA6 7YT
0870 401 7711

Bliss
68 South Lambert Road
London SW8 1RL
0500 618140
www.bliss.org.uk
support for parents of premature babies

Breastfeeding Network
PO Box 11126, Paisley PA2 8YB
Tel 0870 900 8787
Information on breastfeeding

Cry-sis
BM Cry-sis, London WC1N 3XX
Tel: 08451 228 669
www.cry-sis.com
Helpline for parents with crying baby

JABS
1 Gawsworth Road
Golborne, Warrington WA3 3RF
Tel: 01942 713565
www.jabs.org.uk
Alternative advice on vaccination

La Leche League
PO Box 29, West Bridgford
Nottingham
NG2 7NP
Tel 0845 120 2918
www.laleche.org.uk

National Childbirth Trust
Alexandra House
Oldham Terrace
Acton, London W3 6NH
Tel 0870 444 8708
Helpline for breastfeeding and postnatal
problems

National Eczema Society
Hill House
Highgate Hill, London N19 5NA
Tel: 0870 241 3604
www.eczema.org

St John Ambulance
27 St Johns Lane, London EC1M 4BU
08700 10 49 50
www.sja.org.uk
Information on first aid courses

Single Parents Action Network
Millpond, Baptist Street
Easton, Bristol BS5 0YJ
0117 9514231
www.spanuk.org.uk

**Twins and Multiple Birth Association
(TAMBA)**
2 The Willows
Gardner Road
Guildford, Surrey GU1 4PG
Tel 0870 770 3305
www.tamba.org.uk

Women's Environmental Network
PO Box 30626, London E1 1TZ
Tel: 020 7481 9004
www.wen.org.uk
For information on using real nappies

USA
**American Holistic Medical
Association**
12101 Menaul Blvd, NE, Suite C
Alberquerque NM 87112
Tel: 0505 292 7788
www.holisticmedicine.org

La Leche League
PO Box 4079, Schaumburg
Ilinois 60168-4079
Tel: 0847 519 7730
www.lalecheleague.org

**National Organization of Mothers of
Twins**
PO Box 700860, Plymouth
Michigan 48170-0955
www.nomotc.org

CANADA
La Leche League
12050 Main Street W
PO Box 700, Winchester
Ontario K0C 2KP
Tel: 613 774 1842
www.lalecheleague.org

Multiple Births Canada
PO Box 432, Wasaga Beach
Ontario

L9Z 1Z4
Tel: 705 429 0901
www.multiplebirthscanada.org

AUSTRALIA
Austprem
www.austprem.org.au
Internet-based support for parents of
preterm babies

Australian Breastfeeding Association
1818 Malvern Road
East Malvern
Victoria 3145
www.breastfeeding.asn.au
Telephone numbers of breastfeeding
counsellors are posted on the website.

**The Australian Multiple Births
Association (AMBA)**
Po Box 105, Coogee
NSW 2034
Tel: 1300 88 64 99
www.amba.org.au

La Leche League
www.lalecheleague.org/australia
Telephone numbers of breastfeeding
counsellors are posted on the website.

NEW ZEALAND
La Leche League
PO Box 1270, Wellington
New Zealand
Tel: 04 471 0690
www.lalecheleague.org/llnz

ParentCare
PO Box 8297, Symonds St
Auckland
Tel: 630 9943 ext 3223
www.parentcare.org.nz
Support for parents of premature and
poorly babies

Index